Manag n *and Coexisting Disorders*

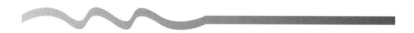

Using the Addiction-Free Pain Management™ System

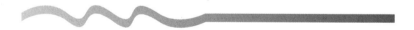

Managing Pain and Coexisting Disorders

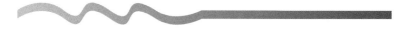

Using the Addiction-Free Pain Management™ System

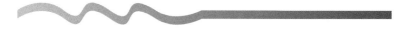

Developed by
Dr. Stephen F. Grinstead

Foreword by Terence T. Gorski

Based on the Addiction-Free Pain Management™ System and the Gorski-CENAPS® Model

This book is adapted from the *Addiction-Free Pain Management Professional Guide* by Stephen F. Grinstead and Terence T. Gorski (Herald House/ Independence Press 1999).

Additional copies are available from the publisher:
Herald House/Independence Press
1001 West Walnut
P.O. Box 390
Independence, MO 64051-0390
Phone: 1-800-767-8181 or (816) 521-3015
Fax: (816) 521-3066
Web site: *www.relapse.org*

For training contact:
The CENAPS® Corporation
6147 Deltona Blvd.
Spring Hill, FL 34606
Phone: (352) 596-8000
Fax: (352) 596-8002
E-mail: *info@cenaps.com*

© 2007
Stephen F. Grinstead

12 11 10 09 08 07   5 4 3 2 1

Library of Congress Cataloging-in-Publication Data

ISBN 978-0-8309-1347-3

Printed in the United States of America

Contents

Dedicated to my father, Robert D. Grinstead

Foreword

By Terence T. Gorski
President, The CENAPS Corporation

When I first started working with Stephen Grinstead on integrating the concepts of the CENAPS® Model with the concepts of Pain Management in 1996, I was doing it because I had seen so many people suffering from pain disorders. I saw many people with long-term quality sobriety relapse over mismanaged chronic pain. I believed that with the proper expert help the basic principles of the CENAPS® Model could be adapted to help those suffering from chronic pain. I never thought I would benefit directly—as a recipient—from the principles in this collaboration; but I have. I believe that your clients can as well.

Chronic pain can be a problem for everyone. I know. I became trapped in a chronic pain cycle that nearly destroyed my life and my ability to keep working. The combination of old sports injuries, a lifestyle of high stress, and the gradual development of severe arthritis and other joint problems left me nearly incapacitated. It made everything that I did more difficult and stressful.

As a result, I moved on to using the principles and exercises in the *Addiction-Free Pain Management™ (APM™) Professional Guide* and *APM™ Workbook*. I'm not pain free all of the time, but as long as I consistently practice the pain management principles described in this book and the exercises in the *APM™ Workbook*, I am able to function normally and am pain free much of the time.

I'm excited about *Managing Pain and Coexisting Disorders: Using the Addiction-Free Pain Management™ System*, which started out to be a second edition of the *Addiction Free Pain Management™ Professional Guide.* I'm excited because it introduces the evolution of the Gorski-CENAPS® *Relapse Prevention Counseling Workbook* as well as Dr. Grinstead's past eleven years of innovative growth and improvements in the Addiction-Free Pain Management™ system. Some of the changes in this book include the latest additions to the Relapse Prevention Counseling process as well as the following APM™ modifications:

- Updated explanations of pain and the pain system
- A section on coping with anticipatory pain
- Explanation of the improved exercise to help clients differenti-

ate between the biological and psychological/emotional components of pain
- The addition of craving and pain flare-up planning
- A revised APM High-Risk Situation List
- The transition from Abstinence Contracting to a more appropriate APM™ Medication Management Agreement
- An improved Pain Medication Problem Checklist exercise

As you read this book, remember—the journey to effective pain management is not easy, but it is well worth the effort. No matter how much pain your clients are experiencing today, if you teach them to do the right things, you can help them feel a little bit better—and in some cases a lot better. If you allow your clients to give in and keep using ineffective pain management and problematic use of pain medication, they will feel a little bit worse—or in some cases a lot worse. *The choice is theirs!* This, to me, is the most important message of this book. Your clients don't have to stay trapped in a never-ending cycle of pain. This book gives you the information and practical skills that you need to help your clients make a better choice.

Preface

Chronic pain is a serious health crisis confronting many people today. According to recent research it currently affects well over 100 million American adults and is estimated that an excess of $100 billion per year is spent on medical costs and lost productivity. See the following chart for the costs associated with selected pain conditions.

Cost of Pain-Related Conditions

Condition	Annual Productivity Cost	Annual Direct Medical Cost
Carpal tunnel	> $17 Billion	$1 Billion
Lower back	$28–56 Billion	$25 Billion
Migraine	$13–17 Billion	$1 Billion
Osteoarthritis	> $8.3 Billion	$25 Billion

Source: *Health & Productivity Management*—**Vol. 2, No 2, 2005**

Pain is disabling for many people, and sometimes there are few safe alternatives available when they are seeking help. As a result, patients end up suffering or developing an addiction to the medications they are using to help manage their pain. Rod Clovin, in his book *Prescription Drug Addiction,* states that in 1999 more than 9 million people reported abusing their prescription medication.

As you can see in the following chart, the numbers have increased. By 2003 there were more than 117 million people with chronic pain and 11.7 million people experiencing either abuse or addiction problems with their prescription medications. Also, people who are in chemical-dependency recovery face potential relapse or sometimes death from their addiction as a result of an untreated—or mistreated—chronic pain condition.

Pain and Rx Abuse/Addiction

- 57 % of adults experiences level 4 + chronic pain, nearly 117 million people
- 40% say they have pain all the time
- 66% expect to have pain all their lives
- 18–34 year olds as likely to experience chronic pain as aging baby boomers
- 10% conservative estimate 11.7 million with abuse/ addiction issues in 2003

Source: Peter D. Hart Research Associates, August 2003

Managing chronic pain can be a challenging process, but it becomes even more difficult when a coexisting addictive disorder is also present. Historically, pain disorders and addictive disorders have been treated as separate issues. Pain clinics experience immense success in treating many chronic pain conditions. Chemical dependency treatment is successful in treating addictive disorders. However, the effectiveness of either one of these modalities is considerably reduced when the person is suffering from both conditions, as well as other coexisting problems that occur as a direct result of the pain and/or addictive disorder.

I personally have seen many recovering people relapse and even die as a result of a chronic pain condition that was neglected or ineffectively treated. As someone with personal experience of chronic pain, I became committed to finding a solution to this challenge. As a result, I have spent the past eleven years developing and updating the Addiction-Free Pain Management™ (APM™) system. The goal of this book is to disseminate what I have learned since the *Addiction-Free Pain Management™ Professional Guide* was published in 1999.

Determining the outcome of treatment for chronic pain with a coexisting addictive disorder is complex due to what I have termed the Addiction Pain Syndrome. You have an opportunity to explore this syndrome in the first chapter. I do not believe it is enough for patients to achieve *only* abstinence from inappropriate medication. Effective treatment for someone with an addictive disorder and chronic pain requires a three-part approach: (1) a medication management plan—developed in consultation with an addiction medicine specialist; (2) a cognitive-behavioral treatment plan—which addresses the psychological/emotional components of pain and support in changing self-defeating behaviors; and (3) a nonpharmacological pain management plan—which includes a tool box of safer chemical-free ways to manage chronic pain and pain flare-ups. The Addiction-Free Pain Management™ system is a strategic combination of all three components working together utilizing a multidisciplinary and integrated pain management approach.

Recovery and avoiding relapse is possible if the patient is willing to do the footwork and follow this plan using a collaborative multidisciplinary treatment team. With the proper treatment plan and positive support, patients with chronic pain and coexisting disorders can have successful treatment outcomes. They can become proactive participants in their healing process instead of being a passive recipient (i.e., victim). This shift allows pain patients to become empowered and enables them to experience a better quality of life.

Acknowledgments

This book became necessary after I revised the original *APM™ Workbook* that was published in 1997. I have also incorporated advances in the APM™ system since the *APM™ Professional Guide* was first published in 1999.

I want to thank Terence T. Gorski, president of the Gorski-CEN-APS® Corporation, for his generosity in allowing me to adapt the Relapse Prevention Counseling (RPC) model for use with people living with chronic pain and coexisting addictive disorders. Mr. Gorski's RPC model has also evolved since the *APM™ Professional Guide* was first published, and those changes are reflected in this book as well. I also want to thank Mr. Gorski for his mentoring and friendship over the years.

This book would not be possible without several major contributors:

- All of the pain patients that I have been fortunate enough to work with since the first edition of the *APM™ Workbook* came out in 1997.
- All of the healthcare professionals who attended my Addiction-Free Pain Management™ trainings and/or use my APM™ books with their own patients and provided me with their valuable feedback.
- One of the healthcare professionals I want to single out for special thanks is Dr. Jennifer Messier. Dr. Messier not only uses my work but she has been APM™ certified and has also assisted me in conducting the Addiction-Free Pain Management™ Certification Schools. Thanks, Jen!
- Ellen Gruber-Grinstead for her assistance in analyzing, editing, and formatting this book as well as her encouragement and emotional support the past nineteen years.
- Finally, I want to especially thank all of the healthcare agencies who have sponsored my pain management trainings, which allowed me to receive up-close and personal feedback that assisted my ongoing commitment to modify and enhance the Addiction-Free Pain Management™ system.

Just as it takes a village to raise a successful child, it takes a team to write a successful book—a special thank-you to my team! I just wish I had the space to mention each of the individuals who have been an important part of the ongoing development of the Addiction-Free Pain Management™ system.

Most of all,
I want to thank my own pain.

I now consider the *pain* I experience as my friend. Without an ongoing positive relationship with my pain, I would not have written this book or been able to share my optimism with those who might be feeling hopeless and helpless because of their pain.

Stephen F. Grinstead
Palm Springs, California
May 2007

Turn to the next page to begin the first chapter in
Managing Pain and Coexisting Disorders.

Chapter One
The Addiction Pain Syndrome

- **Understanding Pain and Addiction**

Addiction-Free Pain Management™ (APM™) is a treatment system for managing chronic pain by incorporating an effective medication management protocol, teaching patients to cope with the psychological/emotional components of pain, as well as developing nonpharmacological pain management interventions. To fully understand the APM™ system, three major concepts need to be clearly defined: (1) addiction, (2) pain, and (3) the pain system.

This chapter focuses on the addictive disorders, the pain disorders, and understanding the human pain system. The following chapter will discuss and define the Addiction-Free Pain Management™ system. Let's start by looking at addiction.

- **Understanding Addictive Disorders**

This book uses the terms *addictive disorders* and *addiction* to discuss what the DSM-IV-TR™ (*Diagnostic and Statistical Manual of Mental Disorders*, Fourth Edition, Text Revision) classifies as *substance use disorders* and others refer to as *chemical dependency* or *psychological dependence.* You will find the DSM-IV-TR criteria for substance abuse and substance dependency in a table in Chapter Four, as well as the diagnostic criteria for pain disorders.

In this book one of the definitions for an addictive disorder is: a collection of symptoms (i.e., a syndrome) that is caused by a pathological response to the ingestion of mood-altering substances and has ten major characteristics. These characteristics are shown in the following table. The table is followed by a brief explanation of each characteristic.

Addictive Disorder Symptoms	
1. Euphoria	6. Inability to Abstain
2. Craving	7. Addiction-Centered Lifestyle
3. Tolerance	8. Addictive Lifestyle Losses
4. Loss of Control	9. Continued Use Despite Problems
5. Withdrawal	10. Substance-Induced Organic Mental Disorders

Let's look at each of these characteristics in a little more detail.

Euphoria

People use drugs because they work—they meet some kind of need. This is true of pain medications as well as other potential drugs of abuse. In addition to blocking physical pain, one of the side effects of some pain medications can be a sense of euphoria. If a person experiences this unique sense of well-being or euphoria when they use a drug or medication, they are at high risk of becoming psychologically dependent and may even become addicted to that substance.

Positive Reinforcement for Use

Recent research shows that when a person is genetically susceptible to being addicted to a specific drug, their brain will release large amounts of brain-reward chemicals whenever that drug is used. It is this high level of brain-reward chemicals that causes the unique feeling of well-being that many addicts experience when using their drug of choice. In this book we will call this unique feeling of well-being—*euphoria.*

Euphoria versus Intoxication

It is important to distinguish between euphoria (the unique sense of well-being experienced when using a drug of choice) and intoxication (the symptoms of dysfunction that occur when a person's use exceeds the limits of their tolerance to a drug). Most addicts do not use their drug of choice to get intoxicated and become dysfunctional. The opposite is true. For instance, people who become addicted to prescription medication at first use it to manage physical pain, but at other times they use it to feel good and experience a unique feeling of well-being that will allow them to function better—or, in many cases, experience the illusion of functioning better.

People can actually become addicted to this state of euphoria. They crave this unique sense of well-being and feel somehow empty, incomplete, or deprived when they can't feel this way. They may even experience deprivation anxiety, which is a fear that if they can't get their drug of choice (or are deprived of it) they mistakenly believe they won't ever be able to feel good or function normally again.

> Positive reinforcement leads to cravings.

This positive reinforcement is biopsychosocial in nature. Biologically, the drug of choice causes a release of pleasure chemicals that create a unique sense of well-being. Psychologically, "I come to believe the drug is good for me because it makes me feel good in the moment." This is called emotional reasoning. ("If it feels good, it must be good for me.") They then begin adjusting their social network to accommodate these beliefs. "Anyone who supports the use of my drug of choice is my friend. Anyone who challenges the use of my drug of choice is my enemy." The result is the development of a drug-centered lifestyle.

The stronger the positive reinforcement experienced when a person uses their medication, the greater their risk of becoming addicted to that drug. This is true because strong biological reinforcement from drug use creates a craving cycle.

Craving

The addictive process starts when someone receives a reward, payoff, or gratification from taking a psychoactive (mood-altering) drug. This reward may be the relief of pain or the creation of a sense of euphoria. Because the drug provides a quick positive reward, the person continues to use it.

With a pattern of consistent drug use, some people come to rely heavily upon the drug to provide that reward. This leads to an addictive disorder, or what is called "substance dependence" by DSM-IV-TR. People need to use the drug to successfully accomplish one or more life tasks. Once people become addicted, they experience psychological distress when the thing they are dependent upon is removed. When people become addicted to medication for relief or euphoria, they experience anxiety when the drug is no longer available. Albert Ellis calls this *deprivation anxiety*. The person is anxious because he or she has been deprived of a drug they believe they need in order to function normally.

This deprivation anxiety then causes the person to start thinking about the drug. *Obsession* is the out-of-control thinking about the reward that could be achieved by using the substance. Obsession can lead to *compulsion*—the irrational desire for the drug. Obsession and compulsion combine together to create a powerful *craving* or a feeling of need for the drug.

Obsession + Compulsion = Craving

This cycle of obsession, compulsion, and craving creates a strong urge or pressure to seek out and use the medication even if the person consciously knows that it is not in his or her best interest to do so. Over time this reward continues to be reinforced, leading to an increased need for the drug. This leads to *tolerance*.

Tolerance

There is a definite biological component to developing tolerance. The increased need for the substance leads to drug-seeking behavior. There are also psychological and social components to this developmental process.

On the biological level, after drug-seeking behavior has been established, the brain undergoes certain adaptive changes in order to continue functioning despite the presence of the drug. This adaptation is called *tolerance*. When tolerance occurs, the brain chemistry of the user actually changes; there is a development of more receptor sites in the brain.

Psychologically, the person starts believing they need the drug. When people start to experience difficulty obtaining enough of the drug, they begin to feel anxious and afraid. Socially, they experience difficulty with other people because of the time and energy they are expending, resulting in *loss of control*.

Loss of Control

The final stage of the craving cycle and development of tolerance is the loss of control people feel over their medication use and/or their behavior while using the drug. The person begins to develop an even higher tolerance for the drug. In other words, it takes more of the drug to get the same effect. If the person keeps using the same amount of the drug, they experience less of an effect. So the person begins using more of the medication or seeking out stronger drugs, including alcohol, that will give the same, or better, reinforcing effect.

At times the medication and/or other drugs are taken in such large quantities that the person becomes intoxicated or dysfunctional. This dysfunction creates biopsychosocial life problems. At this point, if the person stops using the drug, they will experience uncomfortable physical and emotional problems. This leads to lowered motivation to stop the drug use.

Withdrawal

Withdrawal is marked by the development of a specific clinical syndrome upon the cessation of medication use. In some cases patients may use the same or a similar drug to relieve or avoid the withdrawal syndrome.

> Withdrawal as Negative Reinforcement
> (Mental Anguish or Dysphoria)

Once tolerance and loss of control take place, further abnormalities occur in the brain when drugs are removed. In other words, the brain loses it capacity to function normally when drugs are not present.

- Low-grade abstinence-based brain dysfunction is distinct and different from the traditional acute withdrawal syndromes.
- Low-grade abstinence-based brain dysfunction is marked by feelings of discomfort, increased cravings, and difficulty finding gratification from other behaviors.
- Low-grade abstinence-based brain dysfunction creates a desire to avoid the unpleasant sensations that occur in abstinence.
- The desire to avoid painful stimuli is called *negative reinforcement.*

> - People who experience biological reinforcement are more likely to use drugs regularly and heavily.
> - People who use drugs regularly and heavily are more likely to develop an addictive disorder.

Inability to Abstain

As a result of experiences created by biological reinforcement and high tolerance, patients come to believe their drug of choice is good for them and will magically fix them or make them better. They start to develop an addictive belief system. They come to view people who support their drug use as friends and people who fail to support it as their enemies.

```
┌─────────────────────────────────────────┐
│              Addictive Beliefs            │
└─────────────────────────────────────────┘
```

At this point the person is experiencing both positive and negative reinforcement to keep using. If they continue to use, they experience euphoria and pain relief. This occurs because the brain releases large amounts of *reward chemicals* when they use their drug of choice. At this point they are totally unable and/or unwilling to adhere to the medication management plan they agreed to follow with their healthcare provider.

If they stop using, they experience dysphoria or pain and suffering. They start to experience a sense of anhedonia that is marked by a low-grade agitated depression and the inability to experience pleasure. They begin to believe they have no choice but to keep using their drug of choice.

Addiction-Centered Lifestyle

An *addiction-centered lifestyle* develops when the person attracts and is attracted to other individuals who share strong positive attitudes toward the continued use of drugs (i.e., the problematic pain medication). These people usually have enabling support systems that condone and encourage their continued use. They become immersed in an addiction-centered system.

Addictive Lifestyle Losses

Addicted people distance themselves from those who support sobriety or effective medication management and surround themselves with people who support problematic medication use and/or alcohol and other drug use. The pattern of biological reinforcement has motivated them to build a belief system and lifestyle that supports heavy and regular use.

```
┌─────────────────────────────────────────┐
│        A Pattern of Heavy and Regular Use │
└─────────────────────────────────────────┘
```

Such people are now in a position where they will voluntarily use larger amounts with greater frequency until progressive addiction and the accompanying physical, psychological, and social degeneration occur. Their lives become unbearable and unmanageable. They start experiencing a downward spiral of problems—*addictive lifestyle losses*.

Continued Use Despite Problems

Unfortunately, this downward spiral leads to continued drug use despite the consequences. This inability to control drug use causes problems. The problems cause pain. The pain activates a craving. The craving drives people to start using the drug to get the relief they believe they need.

As a result, when addicted people experience adverse consequences from their addiction, these consequences cause cravings instead of correction. As a result, addicted people keep using drugs to gain the immediate reward or relief despite experiencing serious life problems.

Substance-Induced Organic Mental Disorders

The progressive damage of pain medication and/or alcohol and other drugs on the brain create growing problems with judgment and impulse control. As a result, behavior begins to spiral out of control. The cognitive capacities needed to think abstractly about the problem have also been impaired, and the addicted person is locked into a pattern marked by denial and circular systems of reasoning. There will be more about denial in a later chapter.

> Progressive neurological and
> neuropsychological impairments
> will lead to denial.

At this stage addicted people are unable to recognize the pattern of problems related to their drug of choice. When problems do occur, they begin to experience physical, psychological, and social deterioration. Unless they develop an unexpected insight or are confronted by a motivational crisis or by concerned people in their life, the progressive problems are likely to continue until serious damage results.

- **Defining Misunderstood Terms**

There needs to be clarification when choosing words to describe people on long-term pain medication use. Many patients are identified or labeled as "addicts" when in fact they are definitely not. To help clarify this issue a consensus document was developed in 2004 by the American Academy of Pain Medicine, the American Pain Society, and the American Society of Addiction Medicine. They agreed on the following definitions for addiction, physical dependence, tolerance, and pseudoaddiction.

Addiction

Addiction is a primary, chronic, neurobiological disease with genetic, psychosocial, and environmental factors influencing its development and manifestations. It is characterized by behaviors that include one or more of the following: impaired control over drug use, compulsive use, continued use despite harm, and craving.

Physical Dependence

Physical dependence is a state of adaptation that is manifested by a drug class-specific withdrawal syndrome that can be produced by abrupt cessation, rapid dose reduction, decreasing blood level of the drug, and/or administration of an antagonist.

Tolerance

Tolerance is a state of adaptation where exposure to a drug induces changes resulting in a diminution (lessening) of one or more of the drug's effects over time.

Addiction versus Pseudoaddiction

Pseudoaddiction

The term pseudoaddiction has developed over the past several years in an attempt to explain and understand how some chronic pain patients exhibit many red flags that look like addiction. Pseudoaddiction is a term used to describe patient behaviors that may occur when pain is undertreated. Patients with unrelieved pain may become focused on obtaining medications, may *clock watch*, and may otherwise seem inappropriately *drug seeking*. Even such behaviors as illicit drug use and deception can occur in the patient's efforts to obtain relief. Pseudoaddiction can be distinguished from true addiction in that the behaviors resolve when the pain is effectively treated.

Pseudotolerance

Dr. William W. Deardorff (2004) advocates the importance of differentiating tolerance (described previously) and pseudotolerance. He describes pseudotolerance as the need to increase dosage that is not due to tolerance but due to other factors such as changes in the disease, inadequate pain relief, change in other medication, increased physical activity, drug interactions, lack of compliance, etc. Patient behavior indicative of pseudotolerance may include drug seeking, *clock watching* for dosing, and even illicit drug use in an effort to obtain relief. Like pseudoaddiction, pseudotolerance can be distinguished from tolerance in that the behaviors resolve once the pain is effectively treated.

In addition to understanding addictive disorders, pain patients must also understand what pain is and the biopsychosocial processes that influence it in order to efficiently use the APM™ clinical system.

• **Understanding Pain Disorders**

An Overview of the Biopsychosocial Components of Pain

To understand pain management it is important to understand the concept of pain. Pain is a signal from the body to the brain that communicates that something is wrong. There are three components of pain—biological, psychological, and social/cultural.

Deardorff (2004) emphasizes that pain is not easy to define. But in 1979 the International Association for the Study of Pain (IASP) published its first working definition of pain: "An unpleasant sensory and emotional experience associated with actual or potential tissue damage, or described in terms of such damage."

This definition was reaffirmed in 1994 along with an extensive footnote discussion regarding its implications. The IASP definition acknowledges that, for most people, tissue damage is the "gold standard" by which pain is understood. However, the definition

25

also recognizes that pain may occur in the absence of tissue damage and is impacted by emotional (psychological) factors. In a footnote explaining the definition, the authors point out that pain is not equivalent to the process by which the signal of tissue damage is passed through the nervous system to the brain (this is called nociception); rather, pain is always a psychological state that cannot be reduced to objective signs. In other words, pain is always subjective.

> Pain is a signal from the body to the brain
> that communicates that something is wrong.

Pain is a total biopsychosocial experience. A person hurts physically. They psychologically respond to the pain by thinking, feeling, and acting. They think about the pain and try to figure out what is causing it and why they are hurting. They experience emotional reactions to the pain and may get angry, frightened, or frustrated. They will talk about their pain with family, friends, and coworkers who help them develop a social and cultural context for assigning meaning to their personal pain experience, which leads to taking appropriate action.

The Gate-Control Theory of Pain

The *gate-control theory of pain* was developed originally by Melzack and Wall in the early 1960s. It changed the way pain perception was viewed. The basis of this theory is that physical pain is not a direct result of the activation of pain receptor neurons, but rather its perception is modulated by the interaction between different neurons. This theory also proposes that cognitive and emotional factors influence the perception of pain—there are more than just physiological factors involved.

How This Theory of Chronic Pain Works

The brain commonly blocks out sensations it knows are not dangerous, such as the discomfort of tight-fitting shoes put on in the morning then feeling OK a short time later. A similar process is at work when processing moderately painful experiences.

26

In the gate-control theory, the experience of pain depends on a complex interplay of two systems as they each process pain signals in their own way. Upon injury, pain messages originate in nerves associated with the damaged tissue, flow along the peripheral nerves to the spinal cord, and then on up to the brain.

In the gate-control theory, before the pain messages can reach the brain, they encounter *nerve gates* in the spinal cord that open or close depending on a number of factors (including instructions coming from the brain). When the gates are open, pain messages *get through* more or less easily and pain can be intense. When the gates close, pain messages are prevented from reaching the brain and pain may not even be experienced. The gate-control theory attempts to explain the experience of pain (including psychological factors) on a physiological level.

Deardorff (2004) states that when working with chronic pain patients, it is important to carefully explain the gate-control theory of pain along with simple-to-understand examples. This provides an excellent foundation to discuss what factors can open and close the spinal nerve gates. An in-depth explanation of the gate-control theory is beyond the scope of this book. For additional information, please refer to the reference list in the Appendix of this book under Melzack and Wall (1965 and 1982) and Deardorff (1997 and 2004).

Three Essential Levels of Pain Management

Successful pain management systematically approaches the treatment of pain at three levels (bio-psycho-social) simultaneously. This means using physical treatments to reduce the intensity of the physical pain. It also means using psychological treatments to identify and change the thoughts, feelings, and behaviors that are making the pain more intense or distressing and replacing them with positive thinking, as well as using feeling and behavior management skills that can reduce the intensity of the pain.

Therefore, effective pain management must involve not only the patient, but also the significant people in their life who can help them develop a social and cultural context to experience their pain in a way that reduces suffering.

Biological pain is a signal that something is going wrong with the body. The biological, or physical, pain sensations are critical to human survival. Without pain, people would have no way of knowing that something was wrong with their body. They would be unable to take action to correct the problem or deal with the situation that is causing the pain.

Psychological pain results from the meaning that the individual assigns to the pain signal. The psychological symptoms include both the cognitive (thinking changes) and emotional (uncomfortable feelings) that often lead to suffering. Most people are not able to differentiate between the physical and psychological. All they know is, "I hurt." For effective pain management, patients need to learn all they can about their pain.

Social and cultural pain results from the social and cultural meaning assigned by other people to the pain the patient is experiencing, and whether or not the pain is recognized as being severe enough to warrant a socially-approved sick/injured role. These three components determine whether the signal from the body to the brain is interpreted as pain or suffering.

Imagine the following vignette: Bob is his college's star football player. In the previous week's homecoming game Bob scored the winning touchdown but broke his arm in the process. This week Bob is sitting on the bench with a cast on his arm that everyone has signed. This cast and how he earned it are seen as an honorable reason for him to be sitting on the bench instead of being out on the field helping his team. But, in that same game, Karl, a big hulking lineman, "tweaked" his back and was also sitting on the bench. Unlike Bob, Karl doesn't have an observable injury, and people keep asking him why he isn't out on the field helping his team. Karl is much more apt to experience shame/guilt than Bob, which will probably amplify his pain symptoms.

Pain versus Suffering

The psychological meaning that the individual assigns to the physical pain signal will determine whether they simply feel pain ("Ouch, this hurts!") or experience suffering ("Because I hurt, something awful or terrible is happening!"). Although pain and suffering are often used interchangeably, there is an important distinction that needs to be made. Pain is an unpleasant signal telling people that something is wrong with their body. Suffering results from the meaning or interpretation the brain assigns to the pain signal.

Pain is "biopsychosocial."

Biological Pain
A signal that something is going wrong with the body

Psychological Pain
The meaning that people assign to the pain signal

Social/Cultural Pain
The approved "sick" role assigned to people by society concerning their pain

Many people irrationally believe: "I shouldn't have pain!" or "Because I have pain and I'm having trouble managing my pain, there must be something wrong with me." A big step toward effective pain management occurs when patients can reduce their level of suffering by identifying and changing their irrational thinking and beliefs about pain, which in turn decreases their stress and overall suffering.

Because of the two parts—pain and suffering—pain management must also have two components: physical and psychological. The way patients sense or experience pain—its intensity and duration—will affect how well they are able to manage it. The research on recovery from chronic pain is very clear. The patients that are most likely to successfully manage their pain do so by becoming proactively involved in their own treatment process. The chances of success go up as patients start learning as much as possible about their pain and effective pain management.

> People manage their pain more effectively when they stop being a passive recipient and start becoming an active participant in their treatment.

Psychological treatment for chronic pain is meant to supplement medication treatment, not replace it. Emotional stress and negative thinking can actually increase the intensity of the pain, but the presence of psychological factors doesn't mean that the pain is imaginary. Psychological treatment goals are designed to help people learn how to understand, predict, and manage their pain cycles; use coping skills to minimize their pain; and maximize active involvement in positive life experiences, despite the presence of chronic pain.

Breaking the pain cycle involves addressing the physiological as well as the psychological/emotional components of the pain. Stress, which is discussed in a later chapter, also plays a role in keeping a pain cycle going. Stress causes muscle tension, which then leads to increased pain sensation. At the same time a person's cognition and emotions can also amplify this cycle. Breaking the pain cycle requires concurrent treatment of the physiological and psychological/emotional condition. See the following diagram for a visual of this pain cycle.

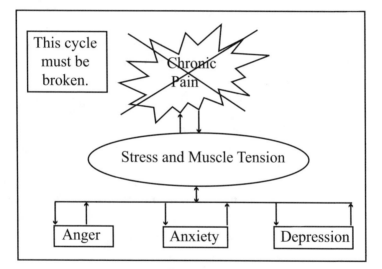

Additionally, psychological treatment for chronic pain focuses on the emotional toll people experience while living with pain on a daily basis. Important factors such as disability, financial stress, or loss of work are also a part of the pain picture, and psychological treatment is designed to address all relevant issues. The treatment for chronic pain does not include magical interventions; rather, it includes a combination of proven psychological treatment approaches combined with medication management and other non-pharmacological interventions that address all the issues people in chronic pain experience.

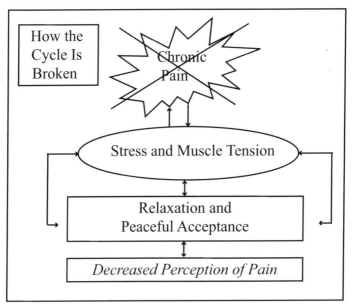

How the Cycle Is Broken

Chronic Pain

Stress and Muscle Tension

Relaxation and Peaceful Acceptance

Decreased Perception of Pain

Because of the two parts—pain and suffering—pain management must also have two components: physical and psychological. The way patients sense or experience pain—its intensity and duration—will affect how well they are able to manage it. In addition, there are three major classifications of pain that need clarification: acute pain, chronic pain, and recurrent acute pain.

Acute Pain, Chronic Pain, and Recurrent Acute Pain

It is important to understand the difference between acute pain and chronic pain, especially when there is a need to manage the pain with potentially addictive medication.

Acute pain tells the body that something has gone wrong or damage to the system has occurred. The source of the pain can usually be easily identified and typically does not last very long—less than three months. An example of acute pain is when someone touches a hot burner on the stove or they cut their hand with a knife or razor.

Acute pain is short lived, but **chronic pain** lasts three to six months or more.

A chronic pain condition will linger long after the initial injury, sometimes for years. In many cases chronic pain no longer serves a useful purpose. To be considered a chronic pain condition, the symptoms should continue for at least six months, while others look at three months as the transition time. Some examples of chronic pain are ongoing back pain, fibromyalgia, and frequent cluster headaches.

Deardorff (2004) states, "There are at least three types of chronic pain problems: (1) chronic pain that is due to a clearly identifiable cause or process, (2) chronic pain that is 'nonspecific' with no clearly identifiable pain generator that explains the pain, and (3) chronic pain that is due to some type of nerve damage or abnormal nervous-system reaction." He also discusses how tissue damage is a major factor in acute pain but not so much with chronic pain, where the thoughts and emotions play a more significant role. See Deardorff's diagrams in the following table.

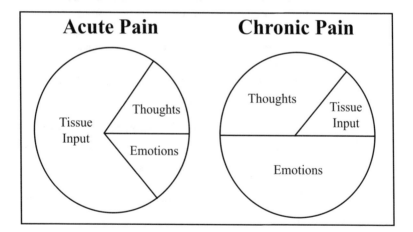

Effective pain management requires accurate identification of the physical and psychological components of the pain disorder. This is where the *Addiction-Free Pain Management™ Workbook* can be used. Described later in this book are ways to determine whether a pain condition is related more to physiological factors (tissue input) or psychological/emotional. There is another classification of pain stated in the following table that Deardorff (2004) calls *acute recurrent pain.*

Acute recurrent pain is when the individual suffers from pain episodes with pain-free periods in between. The pain episodes are usually brief (less than three months) and associated with an identifiable physical process (such as migraine headaches, sickle cell anemia, back sprain, etc.).

The Neurophysiology of Pain

As discussed earlier, pain is a complex combination of biopsychosocial phenomena. In this section you are exposed to the work of Dr. Mark Stanford (1998) in order to better understand the neurophysiology of pain.

Let's start by examining the word *neurophysiology*. "Neuro" refers to the nerves or more precisely how the actions of the brain and nerves are involved in the pain response. The word "physiology" refers to the physical aspects of pain, or more precisely, how the total human organism responds and adapts to pain.

This section will give you an accurate yet easy-to-understand model for explaining the complex biopsychosocial symptoms that chronic pain patients experience. It will also prepare you to understand why many of the treatment methodologies described later in this book are both necessary and effective.

Despite a significant effort to simplify this section, the information covered is rather complex. Our goal is not to describe the technical details of pain neurophysiology, but to present some basic theories and concepts that form the basis of many current pain management approaches.

Pain as a Signal That Communicates Information

The easiest way to understand pain is to recognize that every time we feel pain our body is attempting to tell us that something is wrong. Pain sensations are critical to human survival. Without pain we would have no way of knowing that something was wrong with our body. So without pain we would be unable to take action to correct the problem or situation that is causing the pain.

What is your pain trying to tell you?

Whenever a patient is experiencing pain, it is always appropriate to ask: "What do you think your pain is trying to tell you?" The pain may be trying to tell them something is wrong and they should find out what it is and fix it.

To understand the language of pain, healthcare providers must learn to listen to how pain echoes and reverberates between the physical, psychological, and social dimensions of the human condition. Pain is truly a total human experience that affects all aspects of human functioning.

• Understanding the Pain System

Every human being has a pain system that is a combination of pain receptors and pain circuits. As we continue, it may be useful to refer to the following Pain System Diagram. This diagram shows some of the pain receptor sites and pain circuits that compose the human pain system.

Human beings also have specialized and general pain receptors and circuits. These receptors and circuits usually function very well, alerting us when something is wrong.

- Pain is a signal or warning that something is wrong.
- Pain receptors are nerve cells that detect when something is wrong.
- Pain circuits are a series of nerve cells that transmit the message that something is wrong.

Physically, the experience of pain originates in receptors that are located throughout the body. Some of these receptors are located deep within the body, providing sensations about muscle aches, pulled tendons, and fluid-filled, swollen joints.

Other receptors, such as in the skin, provide pain sensations when cuts, burns, or abrasions have occurred near the surface of the body. Many times the skin receptors will respond to the signal generated from localized damage to tissue. For example, a skin cut will essentially cause various cells to produce and release a variety of chemical messengers that stimulate pain receptors into action from the area of injury.

Pain System Diagram

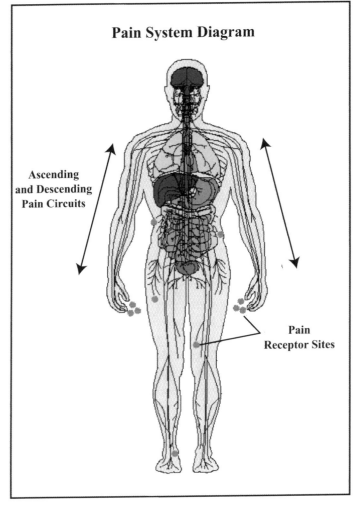

Pain System Diagram

Ascending and Descending Pain Circuits

Pain Receptor Sites

Pain Receptors and Circuits

The human brain and nervous system have *pain receptors,* which respond to the pain where it occurs in the body. There are also *pain circuits* (sometimes called neuropathways) that transmit pain signals from the local site of the pain, to the spinal cord, and then to the brain itself. As the pain signal moves along its primary circuit or pathway, other secondary pain neurons are activated creating a wide variety of different types of pain signals.

Some of these signals simply report the presence of pain (it hurts or it doesn't hurt). Other signals report the intensity of the pain (it hurts a little or it hurts a lot). Still other pain signals report the location of the pain (the stomach hurts) and whether the pain is associated with an internal or external injury (the stomach hurts deep in the gut or the skin on the stomach hurts). Other pain signals report the type of pain (it burns or it throbs).

All of these different pain signals are transmitted into the spinal cord through nerve pathways. The pathways then transmit the pain signal information to other specialized pain neurons, which in turn send the information to different areas in the brain.

Certain types of pain will activate an automatic protective reflex (someone suddenly pulls their hand away from the hot handle of a frying pan without thinking about it). Other types of pain burst into conscious awareness, prompting the person to try and figure out what is wrong.

Specialized and General Purpose Pain Receptors and Circuits

People have *specialty pain receptors and circuits,* dedicated exclusively to recognizing and transmitting information about pain. There are, for example, separate pain receptors and circuits that respond to skin cuts. This provides the ability to recognize and respond to certain types of pain quickly.

People also have *general purpose receptors and circuits*, capable of detecting and transmitting pain signals and other sensations that give information about other physiological processes.

- Specialty Pain Receptors and Circuits
- General Purpose Receptors and Circuits

Because pain is an indication of threat or emergency, these general purpose receptors and circuits give pain signals top priority. When an emergency pain signal competes with other routine non-emergency sensations, the routine sensations are temporarily shut down or distorted so the transmission of the pain signal can be given top priority.

As a result, there can be a *generalized nonspecific response* to pain signals. In other words pain signals can disrupt other systems of the body that are not directly affected by the injury or illness causing the pain. This occurs by disrupting the routine flow of sensation.

Pain and the Cascade Effect

As you can see, the process of experiencing pain is complex and has the potential of affecting all areas of the brain and body. When pain is intense and prolonged, there is a widespread *cascade effect* that results in a widespread disruption in normal functioning.

To understand this cascade effect you can look at what happens when a person accidentally cuts their hand with a sharp piece of glass. The cut activates specific pain receptors, which in turn begin sending pain signals down a pain circuit or pathway. As the signal moves along the pain circuit, a variety of signals related to the pain are activated. These signals are transmitted through the spinal chord to the brain. One part of the brain's cortex receives the information about the sudden pain that has just occurred. Another part determines where the body has been hurt, another part determines what type of pain is being experienced, and still another determines how severe (intense) the pain is.

> The Immediate Reflex Response

While the various parts of the brain are communicating about the pain, another part of the nervous system activates an immediate reflex response. This reflex causes a quick withdrawal from the point of the pain-producing situation (in this case a cut from the piece of glass).

The rapid behavioral withdrawal reflex is a response that is based largely in the spinal cord and less in the brain. Other areas within the brain begin activating the autonomic nervous system, which, among other things, increases the heart rate. Still another part of the brain signals the hypothalamus to start secreting a cascade of chemical reactions.

Meanwhile, the brain overrides a number of routine neurological circuits and reroutes available body resources to respond to the pain. The individual quickly enters into a high-stress response that prepares it to fight, flee, or freeze.

This cascade of effects from the original pain sensation occurs on many levels and involves a variety of different areas within the nervous system. As a result a wide variety of nervous system chemicals are produced and dumped into the blood while other brain chemicals are rapidly absorbed or depleted. Pain doesn't just hurt. It changes one's most basic neurophysiological processes.

- **Anticipatory Pain**

When people live with chronic pain, they hurt. Doing certain things can make them hurt worse so they come to believe these things will always cause them to hurt. In other words, they associate those things with pain. They believe every time they do those things, they will have pain. Because they believe they are going to hurt, they can activate the physiological pain system just by thinking about doing something they believe will cause them to hurt. This is called *anticipatory pain*. Patients anticipate that something will make them hurt, which in turn activates the physiological pain system. The patient starts hurting before they begin doing whatever it is they believe will cause them to hurt. All they have to do is to start thinking about doing that thing.

Coping with Anticipatory Pain

Once the physical pain system is activated, the anticipatory pain reaction can actually make the pain symptoms worse. Whenever one feels the pain, they interpret it in a way that makes it worse. They start thinking about the pain in a way that actually makes it worse. They tell themselves the pain is "awful and terrible," and they can't handle it. They convince themselves that it's hopeless, they will always hurt, and there's nothing they can do about it. This way of thinking causes them to develop emotional reactions that further intensify or amplify the pain response. The increased perception of pain causes them to keep changing their behavior in ways that create even more unnecessary limitations and more emotional discomfort. This can make the patient feel trapped in a progressive cycle of disability.

> My pain is horrible, awful, and terrible!
> AKA I'm suffering!

People's expectations—what they believe it will be like when they experience pain—do affect their brain chemistry. The brain chemistry can either intensify or reduce the amount of physical pain the individual experiences. What they think and how they manage their feelings in anticipation of feeling pain can make the pain either more severe or less severe. In other words, people usually get the level of pain and dysfunction they expect—a self-fulfilling prophecy.

> Patients get the level of pain and
> dysfunction they expect!

The anticipation of an expected pain level can influence the degree to which the patient experiences pain. When their self-talk is saying, "This is horrible, awful, terrible," the brain tends to amplify the pain signals. When this occurs, the level of distress increases—people suffer, remaining a victim to their pain.

But patients can learn how to change their anticipatory response to pain. They can lower the amount of pain they anticipate by changing what they believe will happen when they start to hurt. They can also change their thinking—the self-talk—and learn how to better manage their emotions. They can learn new ways of responding to old situations that cause or intensify pain. As they come to believe they really can do things that will make their pain sensations bearable and manageable, the brain responds by influencing special neurons that reduce the intensity of the pain. The brain becomes less responsive to an incoming pain signal.

There are things patients can do that will make them habitually less responsive to incoming pain signals. Herein lies the rationale for including biofeedback, positive self-talk, meditation, and relaxation response training as part of the pain management treatment plan. In any event, both ascending (pain signals coming from the point of injury to the brain) and descending nerve pathways (signals from the brain to the point of injury) will influence or modify the effects of pain on the body.

> Anticipation of pain affects
> how pain is experienced.

As mentioned earlier, anticipation of an expected pain level (i.e., anticipatory pain) can influence the degree to which pain is experienced. In some cases, when the anticipatory level of pain expectation is lowered, the brain responds by influencing special neurons.

This renders the brain less responsive to an incoming pain signal. This is the reason for the effectiveness of biofeedback and meditation as pain management methods. In any event, both ascending and descending nerve pathways will influence or modify the effects on the body.

• The Pain Spiral

Patients often begin a downward spiral when the *cascade effect* occurs and is coupled with a negative *anticipation effect*. Patients begin to think like a victim; they experience thoughts like "Why me?" or "Poor me!" or even "This must be my punishment." They start feeling hopeless and helpless, which often leads to grief and depression.

This condition is covered in a later chapter, but for now it is important to remember that the cumulative biopsychosocial effects of chronic pain lead to a pain spiral. When people try to cope with this condition using addictive medications, the downward addiction spiral is intensified—although the patient is so medicated they do not notice the spiral. In addition, the brain is attempting to adapt by telling other parts of the body to produce additional chemicals as it tries to manage the situation.

While it is important to realize that pain communicates to the body that there is something wrong, it is part of a healthy defense system. The fact that pain can sometimes be maladaptive, as well, is not always as obvious.

A chart showing another perspective of how the pain system works follows. The spiral starts with the pain receptors sending a pain signal to the brain. This signal gets interpreted as either pain or suffering, which leads to pain behaviors. What the patient does and how the pain system is impacted will either increase or decrease the sensation of pain and distress.

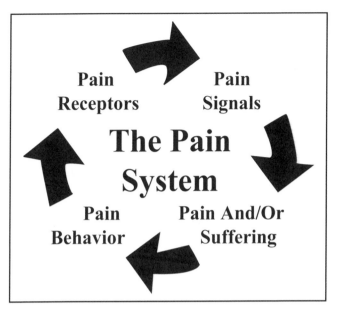

Impaired Pain System Leads to Chronic Pain

As with any sensory system, pain receptors and circuits can become impaired, resulting in chronic pain that cannot be attributed to any identifiable physical problem. The greatest challenge with regard to understanding the biological aspects of pain is why at times it continues even after a painful stimulus has been removed. Sometimes the pain signal gets turned on but never turns off. To help clarify pain further it is necessary to briefly describe the three types of pain.

Three Types of Pain

Pain can be organized into different categories depending on the type of pain. The experience of pain, regardless of the pain-producing source, has the single physical feature of discomfort. However, there are actually three types of pain.

- Type One: Direct Pain
- Type Two: Indirect Pain
- Type Three: Systemic Pain

Type-One pain is directly related to a pain source. This type of pain is well known and easily understood. There is a direct cause-and-effect relationship between the pain source and the sensation of painful stimulation. Examples of Type-One pain include burns, abrasions, cuts, and so on.

Type-Two pain is indirectly related to a pain source. This type of pain includes the pain of inflammation, such as in a sprained ankle or swollen knee, where there is swelling, redness, and the skin is hot to the touch around the affected area. These two types of pain and their treatments are fairly well understood by the medical community.

Type-Three pain is not related to a pain source and is systemic or universal. This type of pain remains a mystery to the medical and scientific communities. It does not possess a clear and distinct cause-and-effect relationship between the source of pain and pain sensation.

> Chronic pain is often Type-Three pain.

Type-Three pain often includes the condition of neuropathy. This is a condition where the pain nerve receptors and circuitry are super sensitive and interpret ordinary input to the brain as painful sensations. It is like putting an electrical signal through an unnecessary amplifier and the high voltage burns out or damages the appliance. Neuropathic pain, in contrast to nociceptive pain, is described as *burning*, *electric*, *tingling*, and *shooting* in nature. It can be continuous or periodic in presentation. Neuropathic pain is produced by damage to, or pathological changes in, the peripheral or central nervous systems.

Since there is no pain source, per se, for Type-Three pain, surgery is not practical and other treatment methods need to be considered. Early recognition and aggressive management of this type of pain is critical to successful outcomes. Oftentimes, multiple treatment modalities need to be provided by a multidisciplinary pain management team. Type-Three pain is often a result of pain signals getting turned on, but not getting turned off.

Unanswered Questions

While the physiology of pain can be explained to a large extent, this sensory experience is a complex phenomenon. There are many theories about pain—such as the Gate-Control Theory covered earlier—but there are still many unanswered questions about the various types of pain sensation.

For example, many people experience muscle aches and pains after a full day of strenuous physical work, such as in a backyard garden. Muscles get tight, sore, and aching due to excessive lifting, digging, and stretching. However, if some light massage or bodywork is applied to this type of pain, the intensity of the pain decreases and sometimes disappears altogether. This example appears initially contradictory in that if muscles are aching, you might think the last thing to help alleviate the pain would be to apply mild pressure through bodywork.

On the other hand, pain sensation will also result when a sensory experience is pushed to the extreme. This means when the pain receptor limit is reached and surpassed, the sensory experience can change from pleasant to painful. An example is when heat receptors in the skin are stimulated by warm sunlight. The results are usually experienced as pleasurable sensations. However, these same receptors also signal a painful sensation if overstimulated (pushed past a certain threshold), such as in the case of severe sunburn.

- **Understanding the Addiction Pain Syndrome**

The final task in this chapter is to understand the connection between pain and addiction. Physical pain is the reason many people start using potentially addictive substances. Chronic medication use plus genetic or environmental susceptibility can lead to increased tolerance as a result of searching for pain relief. Eventually the addictive substance no longer manages the pain symptoms. In fact, it often increases or amplifies the pain signals—a condition called hyperalgesia (an extreme sensitivity to pain) can also develop. The end result is severe biopsychosocial pain and problems.

Historically, pain disorders and addictive disorders have been treated as separate issues. Pain clinics have had great success in treating chronic pain conditions. Chemical dependency (addiction) treatment centers have also had success in treating addictive disorders. However, both modalities often struggle when the patient is suffering from both conditions.

As you can see from the *Addiction-Pain Syndrome* diagram that follows, addiction treatment programs cover about a third of the problem (the Addictive Disorder Zone) when dealing with a chronic pain patient. The pain clinics cover a different third of the problem (the Pain Disorder Zone). Each of the above modalities, when implemented independently, misses about two-thirds of the problem.

Sometimes addiction treatment centers recognize the need to refer a patient to a pain specialist or the pain clinics refer a patient to an addiction specialist. This is definitely an improvement. Now about two-thirds of the patient's needs are being addressed (both the Addictive Disorder Zone and the Pain Disorder Zone). But what about the third zone?

The center area in the diagram is the Addiction Pain Syndrome Zone. This is why I developed the Addiction-Free Pain Management™ (APM™) system that is described in the next chapter.

APM™ concurrently addresses the addictive disorder, the pain disorder, and the addiction pain syndrome. All three zones are addressed—the Addictive Disorder Zone, the Pain Disorder Zone, and the Addiction Pain Syndrome Zone.

Addiction Pain Syndrome Diagram

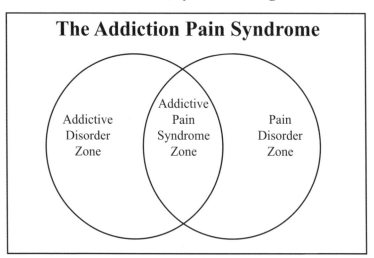

Synergistic Symptoms

The negative consequences more than double when patients experience both addictive disorders and pain disorders. Addictive disorders lead to one universe of biopsychosocial problems, and the pain disorders lead to a different set of problems: 1 + 1 no longer equals 2; rather, 1+ 1 now equals 3 or more. This is called *synergism*. Synergism is a condition where the combined action is greater in total effect than the sum of the individual effects.

Take another look at the Addiction Pain Syndrome diagram, and notice the area labeled the Addictive Disorder Zone. Now look at the Pain Disorder Zone. When these two zones are added together, we have the sum of both zones plus a new zone—the Addiction Pain Syndrome Zone. A new universe of symptoms occurs due to the synergistic effect.

APM™—A Synergistic Treatment System

The APM™ system uses three different types of components to treat the synergistic symptoms, which include all three of the Addiction Pain Syndrome Zones. The first treatment component includes the eight Core Clinical Exercises using cognitive behavioral and rational emotive approaches, which are the foundation of the *Addiction-Free Pain Management™ Workbook.* Second are the Medication Management Components, and third are the Nonpharmacological Treatment Processes. These three APM™ components are described fully in the next chapter.

Synergistic Treatment System
(1) Core Clinical Exercises
(2) Medication Management Components
(3) Nonpharmacological Treatment Processes

Developing an effective treatment plan depends on knowing which stage of the problem the patient is in. It is important to recognize how much damage has been done by the inappropriate use of pain medication and which stage of the addiction process the person is at. Additionally, it is crucial to know what type of pain management skills the patient has already learned. As the person moves into recovery, it is also essential to differentiate which stage of the developmental recovery process they are in.

Historically, addictive disorders and pain disorders have been treated as separate issues. In the next chapter you will learn that to effectively implement the Addiction-Free Pain Management™ system, both the addictive disorder and the pain disorder must be adequately addressed concurrently. Finally, the physical, psychological, and social implications of these disorders must also be dealt with.

> Addressing both the pain disorder and the
> addictive disorder concurrently is crucial.

In the following chapter you will learn about the Developmental Model of Recovery as well as the Addiction-Free Pain Management™ (APM™) system. The next chapter demonstrates how the APM™ system effectively addresses the addictive disorder and the pain disorder concurrently.

• Call to Action for the First Chapter

It is time to summarize what you have learned so far now that you have come to the end of the first chapter. Please answer the questions below.

1. What is the most important thing you have learned about yourself and your ability to help addicted pain patients as a result of completing Chapter One?

2. What are you willing to commit to do differently as a result of what you have learned by completing this chapter?

3. What obstacles might get in the way of making these changes? What can you do to overcome these roadblocks?

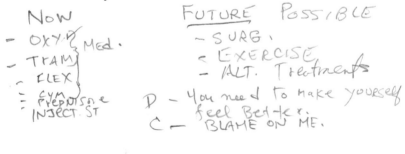

> **Take time to pause and reflect, then
> go to the next page to review Chapter Two.**

The Addiction-Free Pain Management™ System

Once the progression of the addiction has been halted, the next step is determining what stage of the recovery process the patient is in. This is where understanding the CENAPS® Developmental Model of Recovery is very important. A brief overview is included here. To explore this model further, please refer to *Passages through Recovery* by Terence T. Gorski.

• The CENAPS® Developmental Model of Recovery

The CENAPS® Developmental Model of Recovery is based on the premise that addiction and its related mental and personality disorders are chronic lifestyle-related conditions that require a long-term developmental process of recovery. This recovery process is conceptualized as moving through a series of seven stages.

Stage 0: Active Addiction

During the *Active Addiction Stage* substance abusers are actively using pain medication (possibly including alcohol and other drugs), receiving substantial perceived benefits from their use, and experiencing few perceived adverse consequences. As a result, they see no reason to seek treatment.

Stage 1: Transition

During the *Transition Stage* the primary focus is on interrupting denial and treatment resistance. The patient is usually experiencing a motivating crisis, coupled with a failure of their usual coping tools (i.e., the pain medication or dose no longer works). The primary task is to help the patient recognize and accept the need for treatment by resolving their denial/defense mechanisms.

Stage 2: Stabilization

During the *Stabilization Stage* the primary focus is upon breaking the addiction cycle, managing withdrawal, stabilizing mental status, and managing the situational life crisis. For the addicted chronic pain patient this stage requires the development of safer pain management tools while supporting patients to shift from the perception of themselves as a victim of pain to being empowered to successfully manage their pain and experience hope for the future. Other stabilization areas to be developed are stress, craving management, and pain flare-up plans.

Stage 3: Early Recovery

During the *Early Recovery Stage* the primary focus is to educate patients about the addictive disorder and the pain disorder, as well as the related mental and personality disorders. To establish a structured recovery program, patients need to learn about the recovery process and to integrate basic skills for identifying and changing addictive thoughts, feelings, and behaviors.

Stage 4: Middle Recovery

During the *Middle Recovery Stage* the primary focus is repairing damage to significant others and to work, social, intimate, and friendship systems caused by the addiction. For the pain patient this is also the time to fully resolve issues of grief and loss caused by the pain disorder and/or the addictive disorder. It is a time to establish a balanced lifestyle, as well as effective pain management plans and a schedule of appropriate recovery programs.

Stage 5: Late Recovery

During the *Late Recovery Stage* the focus is on helping the patient make changes in self-defeating personality styles and self-defeating lifestyle structures that interfere with maintaining sobriety, creating an effective pain management plan, and learning to take personal responsibility. Since many patients with chronic pain disorders have also experienced past physical and/or emotional trauma, those issues need to be processed and resolved.

Stage 6: Maintenance

During the *Maintenance Stage* the primary focus is upon the maintenance of sobriety, effective pain management, and responsibility. Patients learn to build a better quality of life while actively participating in the developmental life process.

Understanding and implementing the developmental model of recovery is crucial for helping patients recover from the Addiction Pain Syndrome.

APM™: The Concurrent Treatment of Pain and Addictive Disorders

In the previous chapter you learned how addictive disorders and pain disorders interact. Now that you understand how the two conditions overlap, the remainder of this chapter will define and explain Addiction-Free Pain Management™, the overlapping concurrent treatment system that will foster successful treatment outcomes.

- **Addiction-Free Pain Management™ Defined**

First of all, let me define the term *addiction free.* To understand addiction free, it is important to differentiate between addiction, pseudoaddiction, and dependency. Also, remember the earlier definition of an addictive disorder, which includes biological rewards, craving cycles, loss of control, and negative consequences.

Many chronic pain patients are physically dependent on their medication, but they do not exhibit the addictive biopsychosocial tendencies described in the first chapter—this is physical dependency. To be considered addiction free, a patient must be free of inappropriate psychoactive substances and using additional non-pharmacological treatment modalities to manage their pain, such as the ones described later in this chapter.

In some instances addiction free may mean that a patient must take mood-altering (psychoactive) medication, and are able to take it exactly as prescribed. They use the medication for physical pain relief, but *do not* use the medication to achieve a state of euphoria or mood alteration. They do not obsess about the medication or become compulsive about taking it; they are not using it to manage psychological/emotional pain, and they do not experience negative consequences from using it. This is a fairly simple description of Addiction-Free Pain Management™, which will be expanded later in this book.

> Addiction-Free Pain Management™ (APM™) is the ability to manage a chronic pain condition without experiencing the negative consequences of addiction.

- **The Development of Addiction-Free Pain Management™**

Now that addiction and Addiction-Free Pain Management™ have been defined, it is time to look at the developmental process of the APM™ system. This is accomplished by exploring the five developmental stages that APM™ has undergone over the past decade. My hope is that by reading this book you will become a part of its ongoing evolution.

APM™ Stage One: A Personal Recovery Experience
APM™ Stage Two: Working with Chronic Pain Patients
APM™ Stage Three: Applying the CENAPS® Model
APM™ Stage Four: Field Testing the System
APM™ Stage Five: Transferring the Technology

APM™ Stage One
Pain Management—A Personal Recovery Experience

The first seeds for Addiction-Free Pain Management™(APM™) were planted in 1962, but did not begin to develop until the early to mid 1980s. The conception and initial foundation began with an elementary school accident and the opiate pain medication I received in 1962. That one incident and repeated exposure to opiate-based medications, thereafter, resulted in many problems that continued throughout my adolescence and early adult life.

The developmental process or evolution began when I experienced a workplace accident in the early 1980s and realized that I wanted to live my life free of the inappropriate use of psychoactive medication. I was desperate to find another alternative and struggled with healthcare providers over recommendations for operations, pain medication, and physical therapy. We all struggled with the question of "What do we do next?"

One purpose in writing this book is to share the answer to that question. Our main goal is to demonstrate that it is possible to have successful treatment outcomes by creatively combining existing chemical dependency and chronic pain treatment methods along with the CENAPS® Model of Relapse Prevention Counseling and Denial Management Counseling as part of its foundation. APM™ did not fully develop overnight and is continually being improved upon. In fact, it remains a work in progress.

> Chronic pain can be successfully treated by creatively combining existing chemical dependency and chronic pain treatment methods.

The maturing process began with the pioneering work of Dr. Jerry Callaway and Dr. Philip Mac. These two addiction medicine specialists had a vision ahead of its time. They were sure that someone with a chronic pain disorder who developed an addictive disorder due to being on their pain medication needed to be treated for both conditions at the same time and the same place.

Because of my own chronic pain condition and my interest in helping this population, they asked me to take on the role of primary therapist for their addiction pain treatment program. I was now working with patients who had lost almost all hope of ever having a normal life. Some of these people came into our program in wheelchairs or using crutches and canes. As a result of the program, many of them walked out under their own power in a relatively short time. I began to develop my own vision of addiction-free treatment, and the APM™ system continued to grow.

APM™ Stage Two
Working with Chronic Pain Patients

APM™ continued to mature as the result of a team approach that included all disciplines. The basic approach was pragmatic—we looked for methods that worked. I promoted special treatment plans for patients, some of which were quite unheard of in an addiction treatment program.

On-site chiropractic visits were arranged. Two to three massage therapy sessions per week became an integral part of the patients' treatment plans. One of the more memorable activities included trips to a hydrotherapy treatment facility. In such a relaxed and nurturing environment patients were much more open and willing to share. In addition, exercising in water was much more beneficial than land-based workouts for many chronic pain conditions.

> The APM™ system continued to grow with many challenges still ahead.

Within the first few years I worked in the pain program, I noticed many patients who were not in the program—and even some of the treatment staff—began to complain about the "special" treatment pain patients were receiving. Other staff members thought the pain patients were complaining and "drug-seeking." At a time when teamwork was most needed, the staff was in constant conflict. "Now what?" I began to ask myself.

Fortunately, Drs. Callaway and Mac advocated for the pain program and helped me develop a plan to address these issues and facilitate a team approach. It wasn't easy. At times the specialized alternative treatments were not allowed—"too disruptive to the treatment milieu," was the rationale. By educating the staff, we were able to help them understand that the pain patients were not receiving special treatment, but they had special requirements that had to be addressed if they were to succeed in treatment.

> A major challenge for APM™
> was the onset of managed care.

Another major challenge for APM™ was the onset of insurance reform and the initial introduction of a managed care approach. What started in the name of cost containment, resulted in many patients no longer receiving adequate treatment. When chemically dependent chronic pain patients do not receive effective treatment, they continue to overutilize the healthcare system and their health problems become even worse. Instead of containing costs, expenses grew even higher, and some people died as a result of these misguided cutbacks. Even patients who were in our pain program experienced problems, despite the fact they were receiving effective treatment.

Another challenge was that a high percentage of the pain patients were dropping out of treatment at a much higher rate than other patients. During this time I was introduced to the Gorski-CENAPS® tools that one of the hospital's counselors, Molly Burke, brought back from a CENAPS® relapse prevention training. The one tool that made a significant difference in discouraging patients from leaving against medical advice (AMA) was the *Relapse Prevention Early Intervention Plan*, which became the hospital's AMA intervention plan.

We interviewed patients and asked them to answer three questions:

- What are you going to do if you want to leave treatment?
- What should we (your treatment providers) do if you attempt, or ask, to leave treatment?
- Who are the significant people in your life whom we can involve to help you get through the moments of craving and despair without leaving treatment?

Out of these questions we developed a concrete and specific plan of action that could be used to proactively intervene should patients want to leave treatment against medical advice. This plan allowed early identification and effective responses rather than patient management by crisis.

The more I learned about the GORSKI-CENAPS® Model, the more intrigued I became. I realized this could be the way to increase the effectiveness of the pain program. As you will see in the following chapters, it turned out I was right.

Another problem associated with not obtaining long-term success with this population developed after they left primary treatment and went into the continuing care program. Many patients did not last more than three or four weeks before dropping out. Some ended up experiencing painful relapses and returning to treatment even more hopeless than before.

We struggled with the questions of "Why is this happening?" and "What can we do about it?" As it turned out, the answer was simple—but not easy. The pain patients needed their own continuing care program.

The objections were loud, but I was not about to give up, so I volunteered to facilitate the first continuing care group for the pain patients.

> Relapse prevention tools are a
> crucial part of APM™ development.

While facilitating the continuing care group, I learned the importance of ongoing warning sign and high-risk situation identification and management. I knew I needed to understand more about relapse prevention in order to make a difference with this population. I didn't know it at the time, but my search for more relapse prevention tools was a crucial transition for the APM™ system and myself.

APM™ Stage Three
Applying the CENAPS® Model

The big turning point for the APM™ system was a trip to Chicago for training with Terence T. Gorski at his Advanced Relapse Prevention Therapy Certification School. I was very excited when I first got there, but when I discovered what the next seven days were going to look like, I almost returned home. This was the most intense experiential training I had ever participated in.

We attended lectures, practiced clinical techniques in role-play simulations, and worked on treatment applications in small groups. We had four primary jobs: learn the clinical model, integrate it with our clinical style, develop a plan to integrate it into our clinical programs, and learn how to appropriately adapt it to the needs of individual patients. By completing this rigorous training program and the optional competency certification, I learned how to competently apply relapse prevention therapy to the treatment of patients with addictive disorders and coexisting chronic pain conditions.

In going through the rigorous case study process, I discovered ways to use my new skills with the pain patients. I also realized I had to make a dramatic change in my career if I was ever going to really help people with chronic pain. So I resigned from my job and went back to college. It was then that I started researching and writing about what was to become the Addiction-Free Pain Management™ system.

> Addiction-Free Pain Management™ grew from personal experience and the integration of treatment methods for chemical dependency, relapse prevention, and chronic pain.

While attending classes at the university, I offered consultation services for other treatment professionals and started training people to work with pain and coexisting addictive disorders. I assisted one of the local chemical dependency treatment hospitals to develop their own pain management program.

By this time I was implementing even more CENAPS® tools: such as identifying and managing high-risk situations, warning sign identification, and warning sign management. I was also using other ideas that I had discovered in my research of pain clinic treatment programs. I started using eclectic pain management approaches—acupuncture, trigger-point injections, hypnotherapy, chiropractic, etc. These approaches are covered more in a later chapter.

> Combining the CENAPS® tools and nonpharmacological pain management approaches helped form the foundation for the existing APM™ model.

Combining the CENAPS® tools with effective medication management and nonpharmacological pain management approaches was a big step for APM™—one that would help form a firm foundation for the evolving model. I knew I was on the right path now. People I worked with in my private practice were getting effective treatment and avoiding relapse in growing numbers. I could envision the APM™ program in my mind, but knew we had a long way to go. I began to imagine ways to encourage other people to use the model.

Here is where fate intervened. I was scheduled to be on the CENAPS® faculty for another advanced relapse prevention certification training school and had just completed a journal article about my vision of an effective treatment approach for people with chronic pain and coexisting addictive disorders. I asked Terry Gorski to read my article and give me feedback. This interaction proved to be the beginning of our joint effort to formulate a relapse prevention workbook for this population.

We collaborated to design a system that would provide effective treatment. The development of *Addiction-Free Pain Management™: A Relapse Prevention Counseling Workbook* began in April 1997. Again a team approach was crucial to the process. Many other treatment professionals were needed to help the APM™ system through the next stage of development.

APM™ Stage Four
Field Testing the System

In addition to writing the workbook, I also created a training process based on my research and practice with this population. The treatment model was transitioning from a vision in my mind to a real world application for other people to use. In addition, my doctoral dissertation focused on "Managing Pain and Coexisting Disorders."

The more I write and train others, the more I learn myself. The evolution of APM™ is an ongoing process that becomes richer every time I teach a class, write an article, or work with my patients. The process is indeed coming of age. I envision the second edition of this book as another of the major milestones in the development of the APM™ system.

> APM™ becomes richer every time I conduct a training, write an article, or work with a patient.

The development of the original *APM™ Professional Guide* began in December 1997 soon after the final submission of the *Addiction-Free Pain Management™ Workbook* manuscript to Herald House/Independence Press. It was then that Terry Gorski and I discussed the next project in the development of Addiction-Free Pain Management™. He suggested that I begin writing a book that would serve two purposes: (1) to define and explain Addiction-Free Pain Management™ and (2) to explain how to get the full benefit from using the *Addiction-Free Pain Management™ Workbook*.

APM™ Stage Five
Transferring the Technology

As a result of my personal and professional experiences, I know that successful treatment for people with substance use disorders and chronic pain can be achieved. You are all now a part of this journey.

By creatively combining the chemical dependency and chronic pain treatment methods presented in this *APM™ Professional Guide* and the *Addiction-Free Pain Management™ Workbook* you can help provide hope to people who want to learn to more effectively manage their chronic pain.

The Addiction-Free Pain Management™ system consists of eight *Core Clinical Exercises* that can be used with most patients. Some patients also need the *Medication Management Components*, while others need one or more of the *Nonpharmacological Treatment Processes*. Most pain patients need a strategic combination of all three components.

- **The Core Clinical Exercises of Addiction-Free Pain Management™**

Addiction-free Pain Management™ (APM™) has an eight-part core clinical protocol for treating chemically dependent patients who have coexisting chronic pain disorders. We call each part of the APM™ protocol a *clinical exercise.* To make consistent implementation of the process easier, faster, and more effective, the *Addiction-Free Pain Management™ Workbook* was developed. It provides exercises related to each core clinical component. What follows is a brief description of each of these eight exercises. Chapters Five through Nine of this book are devoted to exploring how to use these clinical exercises more effectively.

> External awareness leads to internal cognitive/affective restructuring.

As you go through the remainder of this book and learn how the *Addiction-Free Pain Management™ Workbook* is used, remember one important point. The major purpose of each of the workbook exercises is not for the patient to just "fill out the forms"; the goal is to increase the patient's understanding about their condition and show them what it takes to heal all of the biopsychosocial areas of their lives.

Exercise One: Understanding Your Pain

Many chronic pain patients don't have the words necessary to accurately describe the symptoms they are experiencing. Therefore, in this exercise, patients review and analyze a list of common symptoms that people who live with chronic pain experience. Then they are asked to identify the symptoms that affect their own lives. Next they learn to differentiate between their physical (*ascending*) pain symptoms and their psychological/emotional (*descend-*

ing) pain symptoms. They also examine their TFUARs (**T**hinking, **F**eelings, **U**rges, **A**ctions, and **R**eactions of others) and how they change when they experience a bad pain day.

Exercise Two: Effects of Prescription and/or Other Drugs

Many chronic pain patients use a variety of different medications to treat chronic pain and the underlying medical disorders that are causing the pain. In *Exercise Two* patients explore the benefits they experienced from using problematic pain medication (including alcohol) and other drugs and what they wanted to get from using the chemicals. They also identify the problems they experienced as a result of problematic pain medication (including alcohol) and other drug use.

Exercise Three: Decision Making about Pain Medication

In this exercise patients explore the reasons why they started using problematic pain medication (including alcohol) and other drugs, make an assessment of life-damaging problems they experienced as a result of using chemicals, and explore reasons for deciding to do something differently.

Exercise Four: Moving into the Solution

In this clinical exercise patients define what their medication management and recovery plan will include. They complete and sign a medication management agreement that details their adherence to this commitment. Next they develop a relapse prevention intervention plan that describes the responsibilities for themselves, their counselor, and three significant others to stop a relapse process quickly should it occur. Finally they develop a personal craving management plan and a pain flare-up plan to support them if they feel tempted to deviate from their medication management agreement.

Exercise Five: Identifying and Personalizing Your High-Risk Situations

In this clinical exercise patients learn to identify the immediate high-risk situations that can cause chemical use and ineffective pain management despite their commitment. They are instructed to review a list of common high-risk situations that can activate the urge to use/abuse problematic pain medication (including alcohol) or other drugs and/or sabotage their effective pain management program. They are then asked to identify and personalize their own most important (critical) high-risk situation and write a personal title and description for use in self-monitoring.

Exercise Six: High-Risk Situation Mapping

Patients are asked to describe one past situation where they experienced their immediate high-risk situation in recovery and managed it poorly. This situation map is used to help them identify the pattern of self-defeating behaviors that drive their relapse process. Next they identify one past situation where they experienced their immediate high-risk situation in recovery and managed it effectively. This situation is used to identify new and more effective ways of coping with their high-risk situation. These new behaviors will become the foundation for future high-risk situation management and recovery planning.

Exercise Seven: Analyzing and Managing High-Risk Situations

Patients are asked to analyze the immediate high-risk situation they are learning to manage. Here they identify the irrational (addictive) *thoughts*, unmanageable *feelings*, self-destructive *urges*, self-defeating (addictive) *actions*, and *reactions* of others (TFUARs) that drive their high-risk situation. They learn how to manage this kind of high-risk situation more appropriately by identifying three points where they can use more effective ways of thinking, feeling, and acting to avoid relapse. They are encouraged to apply these new ways of coping to future high-risk situations.

Exercise Eight: Recovery Planning

Patients develop a schedule of recovery activities that support the ongoing identification and effective management of their high-risk situations. They are instructed to write a schedule of recovery activities and explore how each activity can be adapted to help them identify and manage their high-risk situations.

Summarizing the Core Clinical Exercises

The first two exercises in the workbook are data gathering or assessment instruments focusing on pain. Read the following chart for a summary of the core clinical exercises. Exercises Three and Four are motivational with a goal to help patients make better choices with their pain management and develop a plan to implement more effective pain management strategies. Exercises Five, Six, Seven, and Eight are relapse prevention counseling exercises, and the goal of Exercise Eight is to develop a recovery plan to address future high-risk situations for pain and addiction.

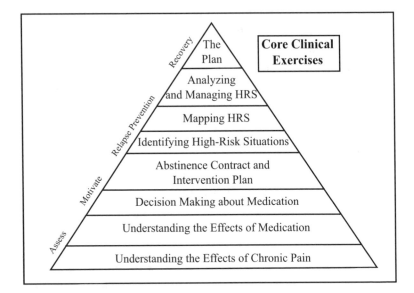

• Medication Management Components

Some pain disorders require pharmacological (prescription drug) interventions. Other conditions may respond to over-the-counter medications like aspirin or ibuprofen. Still other conditions may need a combination of both.

However, some pain disorders can be effectively treated without any chemical interventions. These nonchemical interventions are called Nonpharmacological Treatment Processes and will be discussed at the end of this chapter. However, the focus of this section is the medication management components of the APM™ system. Review the brief overview in the following table.

Medication Management Approaches

- Acetaminophen and nonsteroidal anti-inflammatory medications can be used alone to treat mild to moderate pain symptoms.

- Acetaminophen and nonsteroidal anti-inflammatory medications can be used with opioids to treat more severe pain.

- SSRIs, like Prozac, Effexor, Lexapro, or Celexa, improve mood as well as help relieve pain, reduce fatigue, and improve sleep problems. There have been reports about SSRIs being helpful for some types of *neuropathic* pain symptoms. Using an SSRI and a tricyclic antidepressant (such as Amitriptyline) together may be more successful at breaking the cycle of pain, depression, and sleep problems caused by chronic pain than using just one alone.

- Adjuvant medication, such as antidepressants, anticonvulsants, steroids, anxiolytics, and muscle relaxants, can also be considered for pain relief to boost and/or assist other pain medication.

It is important to remember, for people with a genetic or personal history of an addictive disorder, any psychoactive medication could be problematic. Unfortunately, there may be times when opiate (or opioid) medication management is needed, but there are risks. See the following table for an overview.

Efficacy and Risks of Opioid Medication Management

- Opioids have been shown to effectively reduce cancer and acute pain conditions, and they can also share a role in the management of chronic pain.

- Opioids may be inappropriate for patients with substance use disorders or a history of those problems. If any psychoactive medications are used, providers must take special precautions.

- Concerns about side effects, such as functional impairment and physical inactivity, as well as concerns about physical or psychological dependence, must be taken into consideration when using opioids for chronic pain management.

- Physical dependence is a physiological adaptation to a substance, defined by a growing tolerance for its effects and/or withdrawal symptoms when use is reduced or ends.

- Psychological dependence (often called addiction) is a primary, chronic, neurobiological disease with genetic, psychosocial, and environmental factors influencing its development and manifestations.

- Psycological dependence may occur with or without physical dependence and is conceptually characterized by impaired control over drug use, compulsive use, continued use despite harm, and craving for the psychic effects of the drug.

- What appears to be psychological dependence may be due to pain that is undertreated. This is also known as *pseudoaddiction.*

Please review the information in the following table (provided by Dr. Mark Stanford). In this table you will see the medications, how they work, and for which conditions they are typically used to treat. In addition, some of the other medication and medical procedures to consider are covered in the following pages.

Medication	Mechanism of Action (How They Work)	Treatment Uses
Non-Narcotic Analgesics: aspirin, acetaminophen (Tylenol), ibuprofen	Acts mostly on the peripheral nervous system. Inhibits protaglandin E, a substance that sensitizes pain receptors, and increases body pain receptors, inflammation, and body temperature.	Headaches, muscle pain analgesia, anti-inflammatory, anti-pyretic (fever reducer)
Narcotic Analgesics: codeine, morphine, Demerol	Acts in central nervous system to block pain messages. Activates pain modulating systems in the brain that project to the spinal cord. Blocks signals from descending nerve pathways that inhibit the neurons and thus reduce the intensity of pain sensation. There are many types of narcotic analgesics.	Postoperative pain, as well as other pain conditions
Narcotic and Non-Narcotic Combinations: Other pain reducing drugs	Acts on a variety of neurotransmitter systems. Sometimes a combination of narcotics with non-narcotic analgesics such as Percocet (percodan and acetaminophen) or vicoprofen (vicodan and ibuprofen)	Variety of pain conditions
Anti-Depressant Drugs (i.e., Tricyclics and SSRIs)	Increases activity of certain neurotransmitters.	Chronic pain, atypical pain syndromes

Epidural Injections	Reduces inflammation in the spine (usually surrounding a damaged spinal disc) producing pain. Certain steroid drugs (drugs related to cortisone) contain strong anti-inflammatory properties.	Inflammatory pain from damaged spinal disc, arthritic spinal joints, acute strain of spinal muscles or ligaments, pain caused by degeneration of the spine as in osteoporosis
Trigger-Point Injections	Local anesthetic, usually procaine and sometimes a corticosteroid, is injected directly into the site. With the injection, the trigger point (muscle knot) is made inactive and pain is alleviated.	Mainly used for fibromyalgia and tension headaches. Also used to alleviate myofascial pain syndrome

Non-Narcotic (Non-Opiate/Opioid) Analgesics

First of all the term *narcotic* is a legal term, not a medical term. When used, it usually means an opioid or opiate-type medication. The non-opiate analgesics include medications such as aspirin, acetaminophen (Tylenol), and ibuprofen (Motrin, Advil). These medications relieve pain by acting on the peripheral nervous system.

These analgesics inhibit the production of a chemical substance called prostaglandin E. Prostaglandin E is released in response to an initial pain stimulus. Prostaglandin E intensifies pain in four ways.

1. It makes the body's pain receptors more sensitive.

2. It increases the number of body pain receptors.

3. It causes inflammation, which in turn creates a new source of pain.

4. It elevates body temperature, creating pain and discomfort that goes along with having a fever.

Since this type of analgesic inhibits the production of prosta-glandin E, they reduce these pain-inducing reactions. As a result, these analgesics are a medication of choice for the treatment of headaches, muscle pain, inflammation, and fever.

Opiate Analgesics

The opiate analgesics act within the central nervous system to block pain messages. Opiates activate pain-modulating systems in the brain that communicate with the spinal cord and block signals from descending nerve pathways that inhibit specific neurons, thereby reducing the intensity of pain sensation. There are many types of opiate analgesics; the best known include *codeine, morphine, and Demerol.*

The opiate analgesics are used for the treatment of intense pain. They are ideal for treating postoperative pain and severe pain conditions caused by acute injury. Most people develop tolerance to their pain killing effects within eight to twelve weeks and require an increased dosage. As a result, these medications can be highly addictive. They should be used with extreme caution and are not usually the medication of choice for the treatment of mild to moderate long-term chronic pain conditions.

Opiate and Non-Opiate Combinations

There are a variety of other pain-reducing drugs. Many of these are a combination of opiates with non-opiate analgesics. These combinations can provide the pain-relieving benefits of both types of painkillers and act on a variety of neurotransmitter systems. Some of the common combinations of opiates with non-opiate analgesics include Percocet (a combination percodan and acetaminophen), Vicoprofen (a combination Vicodin and ibuprofen), and Tylenol 3 (a combination of Tylenol with codeine).

Because of the wide variety of pain-relieving effects, the opiate non-opiate combinations are used for a wide variety of pain conditions that exhibit a combination of Type 1 and Type 2 pain characteristics.

Antidepressant Medication

Antidepressant medication may be indicated for several reasons; one is that many patients with chronic pain disorders become clinically depressed. Once again the APM™ approach dictates that a full biopsychosocial evaluation is necessary to determine the severity of the problem.

Some types of depression (situational) respond best to cognitive behavioral therapy. Other types (bipolar) may need a medical intervention in addition to therapy. There are many different types or classifications of antidepressants to choose from; therefore, a specialist should be consulted to determine the most effective medication for each patient.

Another important factor to consider in using an antidepressant is pain reduction. The use of *tricyclic* antidepressants has been an effective tool in pain management for years. For example, the tricyclic amitriptyline is frequently used to treat and help prevent migraine headaches. These antidepressants have been able to provide relief for nerve pain and often result in lowering the dose of opiate medications.

Another class of newer antidepressants is the SSRIs (Selective Serotonin Reuptake Inhibitors). Many pain management specialists utilize this type of medication for chronic pain treatment, particularly for people who live with constant debilitating chronic pain as their serotonin system becomes depleted. This type of medication is good for depression as well as improving pain management.

SSRIs, like Prozac, Effexor, Lexapro, or Celexa, seem to improve mood as well as help relieve pain, reduce fatigue, and improve sleep problems. There have been reports about SSRIs being helpful for some types of *neuropathic* pain symptoms. Some studies also suggest that using an SSRI and a tricyclic antidepressant (such as amitriptyline) together may be more successful at breaking the cycle of pain, depression, and sleep problems caused by fibromyalgia than using just one.

Epidural Injections

Epidural injection is the process of administering a drug into the outer covering of the central nervous system, usually in the spine. The use of epidural steroid injections can lead to a reduction of inflammation in the spine (usually surrounding a damaged spinal disc). Certain steroid drugs (those related to cortisone) contain strong anti-inflammatory properties. This reduction in inflammation leads to a decrease in pain.

Spinal injections are not new—their use in treating low back pain was first documented in 1901. In 1952 epidural steroid injections were first used to treat low back pain with associated sciatica (pain in the sciatic nerve due to lumbar disc herniation). Today, epidural steroid injections have become an integral part of the non-surgical management of low back pain.

An epidural injection is typically used to alleviate chronic low back and/or leg pain. While the effects of the injection are temporary—providing relief from pain for one week up to one year—an epidural can be very beneficial for patients during an episode of severe back pain. More importantly, it can provide sufficient pain relief to allow the patient to make progress with their rehabilitation program.

An epidural is effective in significantly reducing pain for approximately 50 percent of patients. It works by delivering steroids directly to the painful area to help decrease the inflammation that may be causing the pain. It is thought that there is also a flushing effect from the injection that helps remove or *flush out* inflammatory proteins from around the structures that may be causing the pain.

The use of opioids injected epidurally can lead to significant pain relief for severe pain conditions. This technique uses a lower dose of opioid, which has a longer duration and low risk of sedation. However, side effects may occur; so this procedure is usually reserved for serious conditions where the patient is in a specialized care center.

Trigger-Point Injections

Trigger-point injection (TPI) is used to treat extremely painful areas of muscle. Normal muscle contracts and relaxes when it is active. A trigger point is a knot or tight, ropy band of muscle that forms when muscle fails to relax. The knot can often be felt under the skin and may twitch involuntarily when touched (called a jump sign). The trigger point can trap or irritate surrounding nerves and cause referred pain—pain felt in another part of the body. As a result, scar tissue, loss of range of motion, and weakness may develop over time.

TPI is used to alleviate myofascial pain syndrome (chronic pain involving tissue that surrounds muscle) that does not respond to

67

other treatment, although there is some debate over its effectiveness. Many muscle groups, especially those in the arms, legs, lower back, and neck, are treated by this method. TPI can also be used
to treat fibromyalgia and tension headaches.

Two Types of Trigger-Point Injection Therapy

There are two main types of trigger-point injections: injection by
manual palpation and *needle EMG-guided injection*. The manual
palpation type of trigger-point therapy involves the physician man-
ually locating the trigger point by massaging the skin. A trained
physician can usually tell where a trigger point is located, how big
it is, and how deep it is lying within the muscle. However, sometimes it is difficult to estimate the exact location of a trigger point.

Needle EMG-guided injection uses both manual palpation and
guided imagery to locate the trigger point. First, the physician will
feel around for the trigger point. A needle is then inserted into the
area and relays information back to a monitor. The doctor can then
see how to guide the needle directly into the trigger point; this is a
much more accurate method.

Physical therapy is recommended in the hours immediately after
a TPI procedure. Stretching of the muscles enhances the effects of
trigger-point injections, leading to longer lasting pain relief. Whenever possible it is important to refer patients to a physiotherapist or
to massage therapy after the TPI procedure.

Prolotherapy

Prolotherapy treatment is useful for many different types of
musculoskeletal pain: including arthritis, back pain, neck pain, fibromyalgia, sports injuries, unresolved whiplash injuries, carpal
tunnel syndrome, chronic tendonitis, and partially torn tendons,
ligaments, and cartilage, It's also useful for degenerated or her-
niated discs, TMJ, and sciatica. The information in the following
table is from the Web site *http://www.prolotherapy.org/*. As you
will see, prolotherapy may be an appropriate nonsurgical intervention for patients who meet the criteria for this type of procedure.

Prolotherapy Defined

Prolotherapy is a simple, natural technique that stimulates the body to repair the painful area when the natural healing process needs a little assistance. That's all the body needs; the rest it can take care of on its own. In most cases, commonly prescribed anti-inflammatory medications, and more drastic measures like surgery and joint replacement, may not help and may hinder or even prevent the healing process. The basic mechanism of prolotherapy is simple. A substance is injected into the affected ligaments or tendons, which leads to local inflammation. The localized inflammation triggers a wound-healing cascade, resulting in the deposition of new collagen—the material ligaments and tendons are made of. New collagen shrinks as it matures. The shrinking collagen tightens the ligament that was injected and makes it stronger. Prolotherapy has the potential of being 100 percent effective at eliminating chronic pain due to ligament and tendon weakness, but depends on the technique of the individual prolotherapist. The most important aspect is injecting enough of the solution into the injured and weakened area. If this is done, the likelihood of success is excellent.

Prolotherapy involves the treatment of two specific kinds of tissue: tendons and ligaments. A tendon attaches a muscle to the bone and involves movement of the joint. A ligament connects two bones and is involved in the stability of the joint. A strain is defined as a stretched or injured ligament. Once these structures are injured, the immune system is stimulated to repair the injured area. Because ligaments and tendons generally have a poor blood supply, incomplete healing is common after injury. The incomplete healing results in these normally taut, strong bands of fibrous or connective tissue becoming relaxed and weak. The relaxed and inefficient ligament or tendon then becomes the source of chronic pain and weakness.

Prolotherapy works by exactly the same process that the human body naturally uses to stimulate the body's healing system, a process called inflammation. The technique involves the injection of a proliferant (a mild irritant solution) that causes an inflammatory response which "turns on" the healing process. The growth of new ligament and tendon tissue is then stimulated. The ligaments and tendons produced after prolotherapy appear much the same as normal tissues, except they are thicker, stronger, and contain fibers of varying thickness, testifying to the new and ongoing creation of tissue. The ligament and tendon tissue which forms is up to 40 percent stronger in some cases.

69

There are obviously many more medications and medical type procedures available than those listed above, but this was only meant to be a brief overview. One of the procedures described above was epidural injection. This procedure is one of several that are called Interventional Pain Management procedures. See the partial list of these procedures in the following table.

This table is followed by the APM™ Nonpharmacological Treatment Approaches that are meant to work collaboratively with the medication management components along with the APM™ Core Clinical Exercises that were covered earlier.

Interventional Pain Management

1. **Epidural injections (in all areas of the spine):** The use of anesthetic and steroid medications injected into the epidural space to relieve pain or diagnose a specific condition.

2. **Nerve, root, and medial branch blocks:** Injections done to determine if a specific spinal nerve root is the source of pain. Blocks also can be used to reduce inflammation and pain.

3. **Facet joint injections:** An injection used to determine if the facet joints are the source of pain. These injections can also provide pain relief.

4. **Discography:** An "inside" look into the discs to determine if they are the source of a patient's pain. This procedure involves the use of a dye that is injected into a disc and then examined using X-ray or CT scan.

5. **Pulsed Radiofrequency Neurotomy (PRFN):** A minimally invasive procedure that disables spinal nerves and prevents them from transmitting pain signals to the brain.

6. **Rhizotomy:** A procedure where pain signals are "turned off" through the use of heated electrodes that are applied to specific nerves that carry pain signals to the brain.

7. **Spinal cord stimulation:** The use of electrical impulses that are used to block pain from being perceived in the brain.

8. **Intrathecal pumps:** A surgically implanted pump that delivers pain medications to the precise location in the spine where the pain is located.

9. **Percutaneous Discectomy/Nucleoplasty:** A procedure in which tissue is removed from the disc in order to decompress and relieve pressure.

Migraine-Specific Medication Management

Medications used to combat migraines fall into two broad categories:

- *Pain-relieving medications.* Also known as acute or abortive treatment, these types of drugs are taken during migraine attacks and are designed to stop symptoms that have already begun.
- *Preventive medications.* These types of drugs are taken regularly, often on a daily basis, to reduce the severity or frequency of migraines.

The following information is from an early 2007 online survey of *migraineurs* (migraine headache sufferers) and physicians commissioned by the National Headache Foundation (NHF) and conducted by Harris Interactive. The following information in this *Migraine* section can also be found on the *www.healthcentral.com* Web site. The actual survey is titled: *NHF Survey—Migraine-Specific Medications vs. Nonspecific Medications for Acute Treatment*. The NHF survey shows that 20 percent of migraine patients are currently taking potentially addictive medications that contain barbiturates or opioids and have not been approved by the U.S. Food and Drug Administration (FDA) for the relief of migraines.

The survey also shows that patients taking prescription medications not approved by the FDA to treat migraines are more likely to experience drug-related side effects than patients taking prescription medications that have been approved by the FDA as migraine treatments. Although barbiturates and opioids are sometimes considered effective for short-term migraine relief, many doctors recommend against prescribing them for long-term use because of the potential for dependence and abuse and the very real danger of developing medication overuse headaches (sometimes called *pain rebound*). The pros and cons of opioid medication management were also covered earlier in this chapter.

In the realm of migraine treatment, little emphasis is placed on whether the medications have been specifically FDA approved for the treatment of migraine, since so few are FDA approved for the prevention of migraine. In fact, there is not a single medication that was originally developed for migraine prevention. All were originally developed for other purposes. When it comes to treating migraine attacks (acute treatment), however, this is not the case. There are seven *triptans* (Imitrex, Maxalt, Zomig, Amerge, Axert, Frova, and Relpax) that were developed for and FDA approved as migraine abortive (management) medications. These medications work to actually stop the migrainous process in the brain and stop the migraine attack and its associated symptoms.

Ergotamine medications (used as vasoconstrictors for migraine prevention and sometimes mixed with caffeine), such as DHE and Migranal, are also FDA approved for migraine treatment as is Midrin (a combination of acetaminophen, dichloralphenazone, and isometheptene). The NHF study not only involved triptans but also prescription pain relieving medications that cannot abort a migraine. Thus, the issue here is not so much FDA approval of acute medications, but the difference between using "generic pain medications" as opposed to migraine-specific medications.

Some findings from the NHF survey of 502 patients and 201 primary care physicians and neurologists that was conducted in early 2007 are reproduced in the table below. This table is followed by the APM *Nonpharmacological Treatment Approaches* that are meant to work collaboratively with the medication management components along with the APM *Core Clinical Exercises* that were covered earlier.

NHF Survey Results

- Fifty-three percent of migraine patients take triptans as the primary prescription medication for their condition.

- Twenty percent take barbiturates or opioids.

- Another 27 percent take other medications.

- Patients taking triptans are significantly more likely than those taking barbiturates or opioids to report that their medication works well at relieving migraine symptoms.

- Sixty percent of triptan patients reported that it describes their medication "extremely" or "very" well to say it relieves their migraine symptoms completely.

- Only 42 percent of patients taking barbiturates and opioids reported that it describes their medication "extremely" or "very" well to say it relieves their migraine symptoms completely.

- Four out of five patients (82%) have taken more than one prescription medication for their migraines.

- The average number of medications a patient has taken to treat migraine attacks is four (treatment for attacks, not prevention).

- Patients taking opioids and barbiturates for their migraines also reported a lower quality of life than patients taking triptans. They were twice as likely as patients taking triptans to say that migraines "always" limited their ability to: exercise or play sports (35% vs. 14%); engage in sexual activity (33% vs. 17%); drive a car (28% vs. 14%); spend time with family and friends (28% vs. 8%); or simply get out of the house (33% vs. 15%).

• APM™ Nonpharmacological Treatment Processes

Nonpharmacological treatments have proven effective for some pain conditions. Recent studies have shown that endorphins mediate the analgesic effects of acupuncture and placebos as well. Still to be discovered is the mechanism by which hypnosis accomplishes its analgesic effects.

Addiction-Free Pain Management™ uses both of the two components that were described earlier along with the nonpharmacological processes briefly described below. You will be provided with a more extensive overview of these and more nonpharmacological approaches in Chapter Seven. Since each patient has their own unique problems, different combinations will be needed for each. The remainder of this book describes how to effectively implement both the core and optional components to obtain the best treatment outcomes.

Meditation and Relaxation

For decades the chemical dependency research literature has established the effectiveness of teaching meditation and relaxation techniques to patients with addictive disorders. The pain literature also indicates the importance of using relaxation to help reduce the level of pain that patients experience. For example, in her book *Managing Pain before it Manages You,* Dr. Margaret Caudill (2001) explains how to evoke what she calls the *relaxation response* in order to reduce stress and pain.

There are many books and audiocassettes that teach patients how to use meditation and relaxation exercises to reduce stress and anxiety. Later you will learn about the stress-pain connection. But remember, in most cases, if patients can learn to lower their stress level, they will also experience a decrease in their level of pain.

Emotional Management

Most chemical dependency treatment professionals realize the importance of teaching their patients how to appropriately deal with emotional issues to reduce their stress and anxiety. The CEN-APS® Model is based in part on the belief that avoiding painful emotions will often lead a recovering chemically dependent person to relapse.

One of the most difficult and most crucial emotional issues that must be resolved for this population is their grief and loss of health and/or prior level of functioning. Supporting patients to work through a painful grieving process improves their chances of successful treatment outcomes with chronic pain.

Massage Therapy and Physical Therapy

As we saw earlier, direct pressure can sometimes change the way patients experience pain. When using massage therapy, it is important to realize there will be some immediate pain relief and reduced muscle tension, but it will be short-lived if not followed with other measures. This is understandable since there are many precursors or triggers for muscle tension that often resurface soon after a massage session. Therefore, other measures must be implemented that are specific to the individual patient, and these must be used in the proper sequence.

Many healthcare providers promote the combination of physical therapy and hydrotherapy to support patients in learning how to strengthen and recondition their bodies, thus becoming active participants in their healing.

Chiropractic Treatment

Many chronic pain patients receive long-term pain reduction when undergoing chiropractic treatment. Chiropractic adjustments restore proper motion and function to damaged joints, thereby reducing irritation to associated muscles and nerves.

Most chiropractors are also trained in nutrition and many may include dietary changes and nutrient supplementation in their treatment plans. This process helps to build up the immune system while at the same time raising the patient's pain threshold. A later chapter discusses the importance of using supplements as part of the healing process.

Acupuncture

Acupuncture is one of the oldest, most commonly used medical procedures in the world. Originating in China more than 2,000 years ago, acupuncture became better known in the United States in 1971, when *New York Times* reporter James Reston wrote about how doctors in China used needles to ease his pain after surgery. The term acupuncture describes a family of procedures involving stimulation of anatomical points on the body by a variety of techniques. The acupuncture technique that has been most studied scientifically involves penetrating the skin with thin, solid, metallic needles that are manipulated by the hands or by electrical stimulation.

Acupuncture is often effective in managing certain types of pain for three reasons. First, acupuncture stimulates the large nerve fibers that inhibit pain signaling. Second, acupuncture may produce a placebo effect through the release of endorphins and enkephalins. Third, acupuncture may stimulate small nerve fibers and inhibit spinal cord pain signaling. Acupuncture is often used in the treatment of back pain, minor surgery, and other pain conditions.

Biofeedback

Biofeedback is a treatment technique where people are trained to improve their health by using signals from their own bodies. Physical therapists use biofeedback to help stroke victims regain movement in paralyzed muscles. Psychologists use it to help tense and anxious clients learn to relax. Specialists in many different fields use biofeedback to help their patients cope with pain.

Biofeedback has proven to be another effective method that APM™ patients can be taught in order to encourage them to participate more actively in their own treatment. This procedure teaches patients how to minimize or eliminate the physical symptoms of stress and tension.

Effective biofeedback treatment is progressive and includes several steps. It starts with an accurate diagnosis of the problem followed by implementation of the appropriate treatment modality for the patient. It also includes time for the patients to practice situations that simulate instances where the symptoms most often arise. Training the patient to use meditation and relaxation techniques to reduce stress would also be a helpful complement to the biofeedback process.

Hypnosis

Hypnosis can be an effective treatment for various pain conditions. There is some evidence that certain people are more susceptible to the effects of hypnosis than others. The effects of hypnosis are definitely biopsychosocial. Although it is not certain how hypnosis biologically mediates pain, there is growing evidence that it may activate pain-inhibitory descending nerve pathways from brain to spinal cord. It appears, however, that hypnosis does not affect the opioid pathways.

Hypnosis also creates an altered state of consciousness that is usually marked by a slowing of brain wave patterns. As a result, people under the influence of hypnosis often experience a state of consciousness associated with Alpha and Theta brain wave activity. These states of consciousness bypass normal cognitive processes and hence can prevent many expectations and beliefs about the pain experience from coming to mind.

Psychologically, hypnosis may act in the brain to shift attention away from pain sensation. Hypnosis is commonly used in conjunction with dental procedures, childbirth, burns, and headaches.

Socially, hypnosis may create a cultural expectation through suggestion that the pain will be minimal and manageable. The social context of hypnotic suggestion may also distract from the pain.

> Working in the Real World
> with Real People

The following table lists an even wider variety of nonpharmacological interventions.

- Exercise and stretching
- Diet/Nutrition
- Physical therapy
- Yoga
- Meditation
- Traditional native tribal healing
- Talking Circles
- Sweat lodges
- Spiritual retreats
- Faith or religion
- Prayer
- Sleep therapy
- Hydrotherapy
- Healthy avoidance by distraction
- Fishing or other hobbies
- Vocational rehabilitation
- Acupuncture
- Pet therapy
- Sand tray
- Cold laser therapy
- Family therapy
- Biofeedback
- Music or movement therapy

- Cognitive restructuring
- TENS Unit
- Reflexology
- PA/AA/NA-type Twelve-Step meetings
- Cranial sacral therapy
- Volunteer work
- Rolfing or Heller work
- Tai Chi or Qui Gong
- Camping
- Nature
- Beach walks (nature walks)
- Art therapy, e.g., collage, pottery
- Personal trainer
- Sex therapy
- Chiropractic
- EMDR
- Neuro linguistic programming (NLP)
- Play therapy
- Hypnosis and self-hypnosis
- Aroma therapy
- Reiki
- Aerobics
- Humor and/or comedy

The challenge now is to understand how to adapt the information in this chapter to work in the real world with real people. The remainder of this book takes you through the APM™ Core Clinical Exercises with two actual patients, Jean and Dean, whose names and other identifying information have been changed to protect their confidentiality.

- **Call to Action for the Second Chapter**

It is time to sum up what you have learned so far now that you have come to the end of the second chapter. Please answer the questions below.

1. What is the most important thing you have learned about yourself and your ability to help addicted pain patients as a result of completing Chapter Two?

2. What are you willing to commit to do differently as a result of what you have learned by completing this chapter?

3. What obstacles might get in the way of making these changes? What can you do to overcome these roadblocks?

**Take time to pause and reflect, then
go to the next page to review Chapter Three.**

Chapter Three
Building Therapeutic Relationships

- **Understanding Chronic Pain Patients**

People with chronic pain who have problems with, or become addicted to, their medication present a difficult challenge to therapists and other treatment professionals. Pain clinics often fail with these patients because their addiction disrupts the treatment of the pain disorder. Addiction treatment programs often fail because the pain disorder disrupts the addiction treatment process.

Chronic pain patients can be difficult to treat as their pain is real, and they are at high risk of becoming addicted to their pain medications. Their need for relief is urgent. The typical treatment usually involves the use of pain killing (opiate) medications. When treating addicted chronic pain patients, clinical professionals are forced to answer a series of difficult questions.

- What if the traditional medication management doesn't work?
- What if the patient quickly develops tolerance to their pain medication and requires progressively larger doses to gain adequate relief from the pain?
- What do you do with patients who consistently abuse their pain medication by using more than prescribed and run out early?
- How do you determine whether or not someone is actually using their medication as prescribed or possibly not using it at all but diverting it (selling it)?
- How can you distinguish the patient who legitimately needs more pain medications over a longer period of time from those patients who are manipulating for more pain medications because they have become addicted to it?
- How do you approach an addicted patient with a pain disorder who feels helpless and hopeless and maybe seriously clinically depressed because they are addicted to their pain medications and can see no way out?

The Addiction-Free Pain Management™ (APM™) system provides a way to answer these and many more difficult questions that are routinely asked by treatment professionals who care for chronic pain patients. As you saw previously, the APM™ system is a treatment approach that incorporates specific components of the GORSKI-CENAPS® Model. Additionally, the APM™ system integrates the most advanced pain management methods, developed at the nation's leading pain clinics, along with specific and strategic treatment interventions for addiction developed at the nation's leading addiction treatment programs. The result is a unique integration of treatment methods that combine proper medication management with nonmedical techniques. This leads to patients obtaining pain relief, while lowering or eliminating their risk of addiction or relapse.

> A relationship between clinician and patient
> is crucial for successful treatment.

The following chapters will explore and explain the separate elements of the APM™ system by using two actual patient case study examples and by discussing each of the exercises in the *Addiction-Free Pain Management™ Workbook*. Below are overviews of two case studies emphasizing the importance of getting to know the patient while building a therapeutic relationship. In the original *APM™ Professional Guide* I used two of my former patients, Donna and Matt, to illustrate the various APM™ methods. However, since the model has significantly grown since that time, I will introduce two new patients, Jean and Dean.

Remember, this book is designed to help you accomplish the goals described in the following chart.

How to Benefit from This Book

- Understand the APM™ Model.
  –Know the principles and practices.

- Integrate it into your personal style.
  –Make it a part of your routine practice.

- Adapt it to the needs of your program.
  –Improve program quality and effectiveness.

- Individualize it for each patient.
  –Make a difference in the lives of your patients.

As each concept of the APM™ system is explained, you will see how these methods were used with two different patients—Jean and Dean. By doing this you will see the different levels where the APM™ methods can be applied to real people by clinicians working in the real world.

Jean and Dean are representative of the many patients who suffer from the synergistic combination of chronic pain and a coexisting addictive disorder.

Introducing Jean

Chronic pain patients often seek treatment as a result of a complex combination of biological, psychological, and social problems. A pain disorder is usually complicated by other serious problems that need to be addressed in order to successfully manage it; Jean is no exception.

Jean is a thirty-year-old married woman and mother of four children under ten years of age. Jean's oldest daughter found her mother unconscious at the bottom of the stairs, which was the motivation for her family to seek help for Jean. Jean was unconscious because she had taken too large a dose of her medication—Demerol. The family contacted an intervention specialist to conduct a family intervention, which included Jean's husband, mother, father, sisters, and brothers whom all shared their love and concern. As a result, Jean accepted the treatment recommendations and enrolled in a program that utilized the APM™ model.

Jean has suffered from ongoing headache pain since she was a young adolescent. The pain started shortly after she was repeatedly sexually abused by a trusted middle-school teacher. She never told anyone about the abuse. She continues to have troubling flashbacks to those abusive incidents.

Jean has obsessive compulsive tendencies that served her very well in the past. Unfortunately, she also developed repetitive patterns of self-defeating compulsive and/or impulsive behaviors. Because of this, one central-focus treatment was to help her pause when facing a stressful situation and select new relevant responses that can support her in solving problems, rather than acting out old self-defeating behaviors.

Her father is now in recovery from prescription drug dependency as well as alcoholism, but in the past he often encouraged Jean to take addictive medications for her headaches. Like many people who have been sexually abused, Jean has an extremely difficult time with trust and is very resistant to seeking help from others. This is compounded by the fact that her first serious boyfriend was also abusive to her.

> It is crucial to discover the initial motivation
> for treatment and build on it.

Jean's major motivation for treatment originated from the family intervention. She was in a place to hear from her family that she was hurting not only herself but also her children. In fact, her primary motivation for treatment, at least at the beginning, was doing it for her children. Jean's husband enabled her quite a bit and needed an intervention to educate him about the ways he was sabotaging his wife's treatment. In fact, in the middle of her first week in the program, she asked him to come and take her home. It was fortunate that when he tried to do so, another family member called to warn the staff, and they were able to intercept him and intervene in time. You will learn more about Jean and how she completed the APM™ process as you go through the remainder of the book, but right now let's take a look at Dean's story.

Introducing Dean

Dean is a forty-five-year-old married male who has a long history of addictive pain medication use, including alcohol and other drugs. He was also treated in several addiction treatment programs for both alcohol and pain medication over the past five years. In his early adolescence he was molested by an older male cousin and still experiences shame and trauma flashbacks today, as well as difficulty being emotionally intimate with his current wife. Dean acts out sexually with strangers in order to avoid emotional intimacy. His previous marriage ended due to his addiction, having affairs, and his inability to share emotional intimacy with his ex-wife. In his early twenties Dean started using alcohol and several illicit drugs, including speed and marijuana. Dean also has several medical problems. The most critical is a serious knee injury he incurred as a result of a construction accident over ten years ago.

After being confronted by his wife and learning she spoke with his doctor, he finally admitted to his doctor and himself that he was once again out of control with his pain medication; at that time he was using over seventy Vicodin per day. Later in treatment he finally realized that in addition to helping him manage his knee pain, he used the medication to cope with uncomfortable feelings and to get high (experience a pleasant state of euphoria), which would help him forget about his problems—at least for a little while.

Dean also suffered from extreme guilt and shame about having several affairs, which he believes would lead to a divorce if his wife found out. He does not want to lose his wife and is blaming the high amount of pain medication he was taking for making those bad decisions. He would later admit that he also felt free and uninhibited with his sexual partners, because there were no demands to be emotionally present with them.

> Isolation tendencies are common with chronic pain and addictive disorders.

Like many people living with chronic pain, Dean developed a tendency to isolate when in legitimate pain (either physically or emotionally) and would eventually go to an urgent-care clinic. Once there it was easy for him to persuade the staff to give him opiate medication for his multiple physical pain conditions, since his records indicated medical necessity for that type of medication. These visits became hard to hide, so he found someone who was selling black-market Vicodin and his use really escalated.

Dean's motivation for treatment was the result of his wife reporting his increased use to his primary care physician after she found several hundred Vicodin tablets in his work vehicle. Dean's doctor refused to care for him unless he went into an addiction treatment program. In addition to Dean's addictive use of alcohol and Vicodin, his doctor was concerned about Dean's impaired liver functions due to the high amount of acetaminophen in the Vicodin. Dean's use was well over the recommended ceiling dose of 4,000 mgs per day of acetaminophen. In addition to the doctor's warning, Dean's wife, who was working a very good Al-Anon program, also threatened to leave him unless he got help. In the following chapters you will learn more about Dean and how he completed the APM™ process.

- **Using a Respect-Centered Approach**

It is crucial to use a respectful approach in order to be successful working with anyone, but especially with chronic pain patients. That is why I developed the *Formula for Success* process. For rapport and trust to be developed, patients need to feel listened to and understood, be taken seriously, and feel psychologically safe before trusting their healthcare provider enough to fully open up. Before I explain the Formula for Success approach, let's first take a look at what does not work—the *Formula for Disaster.*

Formula for Disaster

The Formula for Disaster starts when a healthcare provider has a preconceived idea of what the patient needs before they even open their mouth. Providers may have a bias or judgment that the person is drug seeking or perhaps being manipulative and they respond from that perspective. In many cases, especially if the healthcare provider is overworked or in burnout, they may come across as insensitive and uncaring to the patient. The next component that finalizes the disaster formula is when the provider confronts the patient and tells them what to do and how to do it—or else! This often leads to a power struggle with no winners.

Formula for Success

Now let's contrast the disaster formula with the success formula. The Formula for Success starts with the provider finding ways to understand the patient and meeting them where they are. This is done most effectively by using a process called *active listening*, covered later in this chapter. When a clinician has understanding, it is easy to move to the next step of extending compassion and even empathy (but never sympathy) for the patient. Next, instead of using confrontation, the provider uses positive strength-based challenge. When all of these components are added together, collaboration with the patient is created instead of a confrontation.

The Formula for Success *A Rational, Directive, Supportive Approach*	
Disaster	*Success*
Prejudgment	Understanding
+ Insensitivity	+ Compassion
+ Confrontation	+ Challenge
Power Struggle	**Collaboration**

• **Therapeutic Bonding**

Both Jean and Dean share the lack of trust found in many chemically dependent chronic pain patients. Many times chronic pain patients have been given negative messages by their caregivers, such as: "It's all in your head," "You need to try harder," or "You're making yourself hurt so you can get drugs." Many of these patients start believing that no one can possibly understand what they are going through until eventually they get to the place where they think, "Why should I even try anymore to convince them?"

I asked one patient why she believed she kept relapsing with pain meds and she told me, "My psychiatrist says it's because I'm a *borderline.*" It took some time but I was able to help her understand that she was *not* a borderline. But because of her prolonged use of psychoactive medication, she had developed some traits that were similar to the diagnostic criteria for a "borderline personality disorder." She was finally able to see that she was *not* her diagnosis—besides, as it turned out, her diagnosis also was incorrect.

Due to the negative messages patients receive, combined with their own feelings of hopelessness and helplessness, many chronic pain patients become very guarded and defensive. Finding an effective way to connect with them is a crucial part of the APM™ system.

Personal Connection: A Crucial APM™ Component

Never forget one important truth—the therapeutic relationship between the clinicians and their chronic pain patients is critically important to a successful treatment outcome. Clinicians are not interchangeable units. Addicted chronic pain patients must learn to trust and rely on a consistent, trusting relationship with at least one reliable caregiver—but preferably a team. The APM™ methods are designed to enhance these clinical relationships—not replace them.

> The therapeutic relationship between clinicians and pain patients is crucially important for successful treatment outcomes.

Without a bonded collaborative relationship between the patient and the clinician, most patients will either leave treatment before they are able to learn about the APM™ methods or they will drop out as a result of the first severe pain flare-up episode or life crisis they experience. Addicted chronic pain patients use the therapeutic relationships with their caregivers as vital lifelines when pain and crisis erupt. Without these firmly established relationships there is a very substantial risk of relapse.

Jean and Dean were both extremely guarded when they first began APM™ treatment. Both patients were defensive and feeling angry because they had been "forced" into treatment. Dean had just come off a major intervention with his doctor and was also feeling very ashamed that he had cheated on his wife. Jean had been increasing her pain medications steadily for a number of months before her family finally arranged an intervention after they found her passed out. Up until that point she did not think that her escalation of Demerol use was a problem—even though she often obtained many of her refills in an illegal manner.

Problem identification and assessment is ordinarily the first stage of treatment. However, the first step with a chemically dependent chronic pain patient is to establish positive therapeutic rapport before exploring problems. One of the best ways to gain this rapport is to just listen.

Active Listening

Active listening is an important interviewing skill that can make the difference between success and failure with a chemically dependent chronic pain patient. Although active listening is a common clinical skill that is routinely taught to most counselors and therapists, the GORSKI-CENAPS® method of active listening is designed to quickly help patients feel they are being listened to, understood, taken seriously, and affirmed as a human being. It allows the therapist to quickly establish rapport and supportively reframe and redirect the patient's thinking in more helpful and positive ways.

The active listening process involves five steps:

1. Ask a focusing question.
2. Listen carefully to the answer.
3. Use same word feedback with an accuracy check.
4. Use other word feedback (paraphrasing) with an accuracy check.
5. Move on to the next question.

This five-step active listening process is used at every step of the APM™ clinical process. The more consistently and skillfully it is used, the more effective the APM™ exercises become. Since this active listening procedure is so important, let's review each step in a little more detail.

Step 1: Ask a Focusing Question

The first step of active listening is to *ask a specific open-ended question* that focuses the patient's attention on the specific issue you want to process. Open-ended questions are ones that cannot be answered with a simple "yes" or a "no." The first focusing question used with most chronic pain patients is "What caused you to seek help at this time?" Another good starting question is "How can I help you?"

Step 2: Listen to the Answer

The next step is to *listen carefully to what the patient is saying*. It is critically important not to have any preconceived notions about what the patient is saying—remember the Formula for Disaster. Listen for the exact words the patient is using, then try to understand what the words mean from the patient's point of view.

> Don't leave "footprints."

Do your best to hear what the patient is actually saying without encouraging the patient to say what you want to hear. Don't leave "footprints" in the psyche of your patients by projecting your point of view onto the patient rather than hearing what they are trying to tell you. It is also important to be listening to what they are *not* saying as well as observing their body language.

Step 3: Give Same Word Feedback and Do an Accuracy Check

Giving same word feedback lets the patient know that you heard them by using the exact same words they used. This helps the patient feel listened to, understood, taken seriously, and affirmed as a person. It allows the patient to quickly bond with the healthcare provider.

> ### "What I heard you say is…"
> (Use the exact words of the patient.)

After the feedback do an *accuracy check* by asking the patient if you heard them correctly. Say something like, "Did I get it right?" or "Did I hear you correctly?" If the patient says no, you say something like, "I'm sorry. What you're saying is really important to me and I want to hear you correctly. Could you tell me again?" Don't get defensive. Don't confront. Stay calm, centered, and accept responsibility for not hearing correctly. Then ask the question again.

> Do an accuracy check.

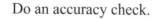

> Did I get it right?

Step 4: Use Different Word Feedback and Do an Accuracy Check

The next step is to make sure you understand the meaning of what the patient is saying by *using different word feedback (paraphrasing)*. Say something like, "I think I understand you, but I want to be sure. Let me tell you what I'm hearing you say in my own words. Then you tell me if I got it right. What I'm hearing you say is…" Tell the patient what you heard, using other words. When you paraphrase correctly, you help the patient to clarify, challenge, or redirect their thinking by inviting them into your frame of reference. You also begin to develop a common or shared way of thinking about the patient's presenting problems.

Then do another accuracy check by asking the patient if you heard them correctly. Watch for nonverbal signs of disagreement. Many patients will comply and say "yes" when they don't really think you got it right. If they say, "You got it wrong," apologize and ask them to explain it to you again. You could ask the patient to evaluate how well they felt understood by rating their response on a zero- to ten-point scale. Zero means you didn't get it at all. Ten means you were 100 percent right on.

- **Common Problems in Therapeutic Bonding**

There are three common problems that are encountered when using active listening with chronic pain patients. These problems are:
- Denial gets activated.
- The one word or very short answer is given.
- The big dump (the very long answer) is given.

Activating Denial

While giving same word feedback or paraphrasing, patients often experience stress and intense emotions as they objectively hear what had previously been private unconscious automatic thoughts. This increased stress can activate denial and defensiveness. It can also trigger or intensify the pain the patient is experiencing at that moment. The patient is uncomfortable with what they heard, so they say things that invite the therapist to become defensive and counterattack. That way the patient can avoid looking at the meaning behind what they said, focus on other irrelevant issues, and blame the therapist for missing the point—AKA avoidance by distraction.

To manage denial, if it is activated, use the following lists of do's and don'ts:

Do...	Don't...
• Step out of the power struggle.	• Try to prove you are right.
• Apologize for misunderstanding.	• Blame the patient for saying it wrong.
• Tell the patient you are interested in hearing what they are saying.	• Give the impression that you are angry or annoyed—even if you are!
• Ask the patient to explain what they really meant to say.	• Keep going as if nothing had happened.

The One Word or Very Short Answer

Many patients will respond to the focusing question with a one- or two-word answer. If this happens, repeat the exact words you heard the patient say. Then tell the patient you don't understand and ask them to tell you more about it. For example, you may ask the patient, "Why are you here?" They answer, "My doctor sent me." You say, "OK, your doctor sent you, but why did your doctor send you?" The patient says, "I guess I screwed up!" You say, "So, you screwed up. Right?" The patient says "Yeah! You got that right." You could then say, "I don't understand. Will you tell me how you screwed up?" This process generally gets the patient talking.

The Big Dump or Very Long Answer

Other patients will respond to the focusing question with what is called "the big dump." This dump is a very long answer that buries the therapist in tons of interesting but usually irrelevant details that camouflage or hide the real problem from view. If this happens, let the patient go through the entire answer without interruption. When the patient stops (eventually they have to stop for air), you could say something like, "Wow, that's a lot of information. I really want to understand what you're telling me. Could we go back to the beginning and take this point by point so I don't miss anything that could be very important?"

Active listening using same word feedback lets the patient know they are really being heard. Often these patients do not feel like they have ever really been heard and were usually talked at, not with, by many of their healthcare providers. This leads some patients into rebellion.

Sometimes patients are so defensive that getting them to talk is difficult, so listening presents an even more difficult challenge. At this point, open-ended focused questions are very useful. Even so, some patients will continue with short one- or two-word responses. The important thing to remember is the need to stay centered and keep asking for clarification. Questions need to be coming from a place of caring and compassion, not power and control.

> The key is asking clear, concise, focusing questions; remaining calm, being patient, and showing the patient you care and are interested.

One of the focusing questions that usually works well is to ask the patient to describe their pain and how it is affecting them in as much detail as possible. If patients have difficulty talking about their pain, Exercise One in the *Addiction-Free Pain Management™ Workbook* is intended to give them more words to help describe their pain. This exercise is explained later in the book, and you will also get to see how Jean and Dean responded to that exercise.

• Collaboration and Teamwork

Teamwork is important in treating addictive disorders, but it is much more crucial when treating chemically dependent chronic pain patients. Collaboration with all healthcare providers is a must for optimal treatment outcomes.

It is extremely important to obtain appropriate releases and to open effective communication channels between all providers. The communication should be approached as a collaborative effort, keeping the needs of the patient first.

> Teamwork stops the
> *splitting process* before it begins.

A major problem that is adequately addressed with collaboration and teamwork is *team splitting*. Splitting occurs when one member of the treatment team is set up by the patient to get upset with another member of the team. Usually this is an automatic and unconscious defense by the patient. This game is called "Let you and him/her fight."

Chronic pain patients have an innate ability to create conflict among different members of the treatment team. This is especially true if the patient really does suffer from an *antisocial, borderline,* or a *passive-aggressive personality style or disorder.* Team members can experience a disruptive split and be at odds with each other unless the whole team is working together, keeping communications open and clear.

Work *with* Patients Not *on* Patients

It is important to remember that the patient is the most important member of the treatment team. It is easy for treatment providers to *work on* their patients instead of *working with* their patients. The best results are obtained when the patient is empowered to be the "captain" of the team and the healthcare providers are "guides and coaches." Chronic pain research shows that the best treatment outcomes are obtained when patients are proactively involved in their own healing process.

> Treatment outcomes improve when patients are proactive in their own treatment and recovery process.

Some patients will present with an "underdog" personality style marked by helplessness, hopelessness, and the belief they must be rescued by the powerful caregiver. These patients must be taught to be more assertive and informed about their rights and responsibilities in treatment. This is especially true when patients have been struggling with their pain for so long they have become depressed and feel hopeless.

Other patients will present with a "top-dog" personality style marked by a tendency to challenge authority, break rules, and blame others. These patients must be taught to let go of control and follow treatment recommendations whether they want to or not, and the treatment provider must set firm assertive limits and boundaries.

When you have patients with extreme underdog or top-dog personality styles, it may be necessary to connect the patient with appropriate referrals, such as a psychologist or psychotherapist, to deal with those obstacles.

Build a Referral Network

Another essential component for delivering effective APM™ treatment is being knowledgeable regarding what resources are available in the local area. Networking with other healthcare providers allows exchange of ideas and referral sources.

Contacts with other professionals can also be obtained by attending workshops and trainings specific to the needs of APM™ patients. Showing up early and getting to know other participants and the instructors allows for a personal connection. This personal touch is important for successful collaboration and teamwork.

How to Build the APM™ Foundation

- Understand chronic pain patients.
- Build a therapeutic bond with them.
- Collaborate and team-up with others.

Once all the above steps are implemented, APM™ treatment can begin. We invite you to become a part of the APM™ system of treatment. The remainder of the book will explain how the APM™ system works and show how using the *Addiction-Free Pain Management™ Workbook* facilitates successful treatment outcomes. In the following chapters you will continue to see how Jean and Dean work through the APM™ treatment process.

• **Call to Action for the Third Chapter**

It is time to summarize what you have learned so far now that you have come to the end of the third chapter. Please answer the questions below.

1. What is the most important thing you have learned about yourself and your ability to help addicted pain patients as a result of completing Chapter Three?

2. What are you willing to commit to do differently as a result of what you have learned by completing this chapter?

3. What obstacles might get in the way of making these changes? What can you do to overcome these roadblocks?

**Take time to pause and reflect, then
go to the next page to review Chapter Four.**

Chapter Four
Identification and Assessment

• The Initial Interview

The initial interview with an APM™ patient is the most crucial point in the treatment process. Additionally, making sure that releases are signed with other healthcare providers, as well as the patient's significant others, increases the probability of a favorable treatment outcome.

Achieving an accurate identification and assessment is extremely important in all healthcare cases. It is especially important when a person is suffering from both addiction and a coexisting chronic pain disorder. Using focused questions and active listening are effective tools for gaining a better understanding of a person with chronic pain as well as creating therapeutic rapport. It is important to understand the whole person, not just their pain condition.

To facilitate accurate assessments, the APM™ system encourages a DSM-IV-TR multiaxial approach. This approach is not utilized for labeling or even diagnostic purposes, but to obtain a precise picture of the presenting problems and to facilitate communication with other healthcare providers and/or insurance companies. This assessment information is crucial in the development of an effective treatment plan.

• DSM-IV-TR Defined

The term DSM-IV-TR is short for *Diagnostic and Statistical Manual of Mental Disorders, Fourth Edition, Text Revision.* This book is developed and published by the American Psychiatric Association. The DSM-IV-TR is used by a wide diversity of healthcare practitioners, including psychiatrists, physicians, psychologists, counselors, therapists, social workers, nurses, etc. It is used as a practical guide for gathering clinical information and improving communication between providers.

The DSM uses a multiaxial format. In other words it gives the big picture of the person by looking at the following five areas.

- **Axis I:** Clinical disorders and other treatment conditions
- **Axis II:** Personality disorders and mental retardation
- **Axis III:** General medical conditions
- **Axis IV:** Psychosocial and environmental problems
- **Axis V:** Global assessment of functioning

The DSM-IV-TR covers the biopsychosocial areas that were touched on earlier and will be expanded later. Later in this chapter you will learn about Jean and Dean's DSM-IV-TR multiaxial diagnostic impressions. You also have an opportunity to review Jean and Dean's assessment information and examine some of their answers to the *APM™ Workbook* exercises.

Axis I: Clinical Disorders and Other Treatment Conditions

It is important to see which Axis I problems need immediate clinical attention. Axis I includes the two primary issues of substance use disorders and chronic pain disorders. It is also used to identify other related conditions such as mood disorders (i.e., depression), anxiety disorders, substance-related disorders (i.e., substance induced organic mental disorders), mental disorders due to a medical condition, etc.

Axis II: Personality Disorders and Mental Retardation

Axis II is used to document personality styles that could sabotage treatment. People with extreme *top-dog or Cluster B* personality styles (antisocial, narcissistic, histrionic, or borderline personality disorders) will find it difficult to bond with treatment providers and cause them to challenge the treatment team, break rules, refuse to accept responsibility for negative outcomes, and blame others. People with extreme *underdog* or *Cluster C* personality styles (dependent personality disorder and avoidant personality disorder) can become overly dependent on treatment and/or resist difficult steps in the treatment plan by using passive-aggressive tactics.

They compulsively go through the motions of treatment without really looking at or changing the core issues.

Axis III: General Medical Conditions

Many people who develop a substance use disorder or pseudo-addiction usually have an undertreated or mistreated chronic pain condition. Medical professionals (such as doctors, physician assistants, nurse practitioners, and nurses) are the best team members to gather information for the Axis III medical conditions. A well-trained and experienced medical professional can gain tremendous insights into the most difficult patients by completing an in-depth history and physical. A highly skilled nurse can uncover even the most overlooked problems by completing a comprehensive nursing assessment.

Axis IV: Psychosocial and Environmental Problems

The Axis IV area covers other issues that could impede successful outcomes such as the psychosocial or environmental conditions, including lack of social support, economic problems, career problems, family problems, or legal problems. A good example of Axis IV problems are the many difficulties that people on disability experience. These psychosocial areas significantly influence how patients cope with their pain as well as their lives. These coping styles can lead to serious problems that sometimes develop into extremely dysfunctional coping patterns.

Axis V: Global Assessment of Functioning

The global assessment of functioning on Axis V is based on the hundred-point Global Assessment of Functioning (GAF) scale. This scale is a continuum of mental-health illness, with 1–10 being extreme danger of hurting self or others and 91–100 being superior functioning. When assessing levels of functioning, it is important to look at all domains (e.g., family, social, occupational) using the Social Occupational Functioning Assessment (SOFA) scale in order to get a complete and accurate understanding of the individual as well as their treatment needs. The SOFA scale is also rated on a similar 1–100 scale.

• Using DSM-IV-TR Criteria

We have examined the five Axis DSM-IV-TR diagnostic categories. Later you will have an opportunity to review Jean and Dean's assessment results. Although Jean and Dean met the requirements for several different diagnoses, the most important ones are the pain and addictive disorders. Note the following tables that show the DSM-IV-TR criteria for these two specific disorders.

DSM-IV-TR Pain Disorder

A. Pain in one or more anatomical sites is the predominant focus of the clinical presentation and is of sufficient severity to warrant clinical attention.

B. The pain causes clinically significant distress or impairment in social, occupational, or other important areas of functioning.

C. Psychological factors are judged to have an important role in the onset, severity, exacerbation, or maintenance of the pain.

D. The symptoms or deficit is not intentionally produced or feigned (as in factitious disorder or malingering).

E. The pain is not better accounted for by a mood, anxiety, or psychotic disorder and does not meet criteria for dyspareunia.

Code as Follows:

307.80: Pain Disorder Associated with Psychological Factors

OR

307.89: Pain Disorder Associated with Both Psychological Factors and a General Medical Condition

Specify if:

Acute: duration of less than 6 months

Chronic: duration of 6 months or longer

DSM-IV-TR Substance Abuse Disorder

A. A maladaptive pattern of substance use leading to clinically significant impairment or distress, as manifested by one (or more) of the following, occurring within a 12-month period:

 1. Recurrent substance use resulting in a failure to fulfill major role obligations at work, school, or home (e.g., repeated absences or poor work performance related to substance use; substance-related absences, suspensions, or expulsions from school; neglect of children or household)

 2. Recurrent substance use in situations where it is physically hazardous (e.g., driving an automobile or operating a machine when impaired by substance use)

 3. Recurrent substance-related legal problems (e.g., arrests of substance-related disorderly conduct)

 4. Continued use despite having persistent or recurrent social or interpersonal problems caused or exacerbated by the effects of the substance (e.g., arguments with spouse about consequences of intoxication, physical fights)

B. The symptoms have never met the criteria for Substance Dependence for this class of substance.

DSM-IV-TR Substance Dependence Disorder

A maladaptive pattern of substance use leading to clinically significant impairment or distress, as manifested by three (or more) of the following, occurring at any time in the same 12-month period:

1. Tolerance, as defined by either of the following:
   a. A need for markedly increased amounts of the substance to achieve intoxication or desired effect
   b. Markedly diminished effect with continued use of the same amount of the substance

2. Withdrawal, as manifested by either of the following:
   a. The characteristic withdrawal syndrome for the substance (refer to Criteria A and B of the criteria sets for withdrawal from the specific substance)
   b. The same (or closely related) substance is taken to relieve or avoid withdrawal symptoms.

3. The substance is often taken in larger amounts or over a longer period of time than was intended.

4. There is a persistent desire or unsuccessful efforts to cut down or control substance use.

5. A great deal of time is spent in activities necessary to obtain the substance (e.g., visiting multiple doctors or driving long distances), use the substance (e.g., chain-smoking) or recover from its effects.

6. Important social, occupational, or recreational activities are given up or reduced because of substance use.

7. The substance use is continued despite knowledge of having a persistent or recurrent physical or

psychological problem that is likely to have been caused or exacerbated by the substance (e.g., current cocaine use despite recognition of cocaine-induced depression, or continued drinking despite recognition that an ulcer was made worse by alcohol consumption).

Specify if:

With Physiological Dependence: evidence of tolerance or withdrawal (i.e., either item 1 or 2 is present)

Without Physiological Dependence: no evidence of tolerance or withdrawal (i.e., neither item 1 nor 2 is present)

As was stated in Chapter One, the description and ten stages of an addictive disorder are different than the DSM-IV-TR criteria listed above. However, as you will notice in the reproduced table of *Addictive Disorder Symptoms* that follows, everything in the DSM-IV-TR is covered, but sometimes different words and concepts are used.

• Addictive Disorder Symptoms

1. Euphoria
2. Craving
3. Tolerance
4. Loss of Control
5. Withdrawal
6. Inability to Abstain
7. Addiction-Centered Lifestyle
8. Addictive Lifestyle Losses
9. Continued Use Despite Problems
10. Substance-Induced Organic Mental Disorders

Below are the DSM-IV-TR diagnostic impressions for Jean and Dean at the beginning of their treatment. As you follow these two cases throughout the remainder of this book, you will also have an opportunity to see how Dean and Jean completed the Exercise One protocols in the *Addiction-Free Pain Management™ Workbook.*

Dean: DSM-IV-TR Multiaxis Diagnostic Impressions

Dean is a forty-five-year-old married male who has a long history of addictive use of medication, including alcohol and other drugs, as well as being treated in several addiction treatment programs for both alcohol and pain medication over the past five years. In his early twenties Dean started using alcohol and several illicit drugs, including speed and marijuana. Dean also has several medical problems; most critical is a serious knee injury he incurred as a result of a construction accident over ten years ago. He had a failed knee surgery seven years ago and blames his need for addiction treatment over the past few years, as well as his current increased medication use, on that. Dean has been alcohol free since his last treatment episode, but admits to being tempted to start drinking again to help him cope with his pain.

Axis I:

304.00   *Primary Diagnosis:* Opioid Dependence

292.0   Opioid Withdrawal; protracted (post acute) withdrawal

307.89   Pain Disorder; chronic with both psychological and medical conditions (Chronic Knee Pain)

309.28   Adjustment Disorder with mixed anxiety and depressed mood

309.81   Posttraumatic Stress Disorder (adolescent sexual trauma)

300.00   Anxiety Disorder (NOS)

302.70   Sexual Dysfunction (NOS)

Axis II:

301.83   Rule Out; Borderline Personality Disorder

301.82   Rule Out; Avoidant Personality Disorder

Axis III:

Right Knee Injury with failed surgery; chronic

Axis IV:

V62.2   Occupational Problem; currently on Medical
        Disability Status

V61.1   Partner Relational Problem; history of Dean
        having extramarital affairs

        Serious isolation tendencies

        Need for a healthy daily structure

        Continuing need for social, spiritual, and
        Twelve-Step support

Axis V:

GAF   =40–50 Past Year

GAF   =50 (current; but fluctuates with pain condition)

Jean: DSM-IV-TR Multiaxis Diagnostic Impressions

Jean is a thirty-year-old married woman and mother of four children under ten years of age. Jean's oldest daughter found her mother unconscious at the bottom of the stairs, which was the motivation for her family to seek help for Jean. Jean was unconscious because she had taken too large a dose of her medication—Demerol. As a result, the family contacted an intervention specialist to conduct a family intervention. At the intervention Jean's family—including her husband, mother, father, sisters, and brothers—all shared their concerns. Jean accepted the treatment recommendations and enrolled in a treatment program that utilizes the APM™ model.

Jean has suffered from ongoing cluster and migraine headache pain since she was a young adolescent. The pain started shortly after she was repeatedly sexually abused by a trusted middle school teacher that she told no one about. She continues to have troubling flashbacks to those abusive incidents.

Axis I:

304.00 *Primary Diagnosis:* Opioid Dependence

292.0   Opioid Withdrawal; protracted (post acute) withdrawal

307.89 Pain Disorder; chronic with both psychological and medical conditions

309.28 Adjustment Disorder with mixed anxiety and depressed mood

309.81 Posttraumatic Stress Disorder (History of early adolescent sexual trauma)

Axis II:

301.83 Rule Out; Borderline Personality Disorder

301.4   Rule Out; Obsessive Compulsive Personality Disorder

Axis III:

Chronic Headache; cluster type and migraine type

Axis IV:

V61.1   Partner relational problem; spouse is very enabling

V61.20 Parent relational problem; her father is chemically dependent

V61.20 Parent-Child Relational Problem; poor parenting due to Rx Use

Need for social support due to major isolation tendencies

Axis V:

GAF   =40–45 Past Year

GAF   =55 (current; but fluctuates with pain condition)

• The Role of Clinical Depression

Clinical depression is the Axis-I condition that causes the biggest problems for most people with chronic pain—and is often underdiagnosed and/or undertreated. A variety of recent medical studies have drawn a strong association between chronic pain and a diagnosis of major depression. The two conditions seem to go hand in hand in a large percentage of unfortunate patients who suffer the debilitating effects of both chronically painful conditions and persistent mood problems. Although neither Jean nor Dean meet the full diagnostic criteria for a depressive disorder, both do experience episodes of subclinical depression that need to be addressed.

Researchers still cannot determine whether there is a cause-and-effect relationship between chronic pain and depression, and, if there is, which condition causes the other. Some research suggests that insufficiently treated, ongoing pain may cause changes in the chemical environment of the brain, thereby increasing the likelihood of depression. Similarly, other research suggests that insufficiently treated, ongoing depression causes changes in the chemical environment of the brain such that it increases an individual's perception of painful sensations. Regardless of the etiology, concurrent treatment is necessary for successful treatment outcomes.

Hitting the Wall Called Depression

There are several types of clinical depression that involve disturbances in mood, concentration, self-confidence, sleep, appetite, activity, and behavior as well as disruptions in friendships, family, work, and/or school. A clinical depression is different than the experiences of sadness, disappointment, and grief familiar to everyone, which sometimes makes it difficult to determine when professional help is necessary. The following information is intended to provide you with a brief overview of the symptoms, causes, and treatment of clinical depression and offers you tools to assess the severity of any symptoms that your patients may be experiencing to determine whether you should consider developing a depression treatment plan at this time.

> Feeling Down versus Being Depressed

A period of depressed mood that lasts for several days or a few weeks is often just a normal part of life and is not necessarily a cause for concern. Although these feelings are often referred to as depression, they typically do not constitute a clinical depression because the symptoms are relatively mild and only last for a short period of time. Moreover, milder periods of depression are often related to specific, stressful life events, and improvement frequently coincides with the reduction or elimination of the stressor.

A person experiencing a clinical depression, however, experiences substantial changes in their mood, thinking, behaviors, activities, and self-perceptions. A depressed person often has difficulty making decisions; for example, the day-to-day tasks of paying bills, attending classes, reading assignments, and returning phone calls may seem overwhelming.

A depressed person may also dwell on negative thoughts, focus on unpleasant experiences, describe themselves as a failure, report that things are hopeless, and feel as though they are a burden to others. The changes in mood brought on by depression frequently result in feelings of sadness, irritability, anger, emptiness, and/or anxiety and may even lead to thoughts of suicide.

There are also different types of depression, including bipolar disorder, where depressive episodes alternate with manic or hypomanic episodes that may include feelings of agitation and euphoria. A severe or long-term depressive episode can substantially wear down self-esteem and may result in thoughts of death and even attempts of suicide.

Review the following information on a depression rating scale for patients. The assessment and ratings are from the work of Terence T. Gorski (2006), *Depression and Relapse: A Guide to Recovery,* and is used here with his generous permission. If you have clients with an addictive disorder and co-occurring depression, you may want to consider obtaining Mr. Gorki's depression book for a more in-depth process that is beyond the scope of this book.

Gorski's Depression Rating Instrument

Please be honest with yourself as you complete the following.

- How depressed are you? **Rate 0–10_____, where:**

1 = When I get depressed, my depression is a nuisance, but I can always function normally with extra effort.

5 = When I get depressed, at times I can function normally with extra effort and at other times I can't.

10 = When I get depressed, I usually can't function normally even with extra effort.

- How often do you feel depressed? **Rate 0–10 _____, where:**

1 = Almost never

5 = Almost half the time

10 = Almost all of the time

- How long does each episode of depression last? **Rate 0–10 _____, where:**

1 = Less than an hour

5 = Several days

10 = I'm depressed all of the time with no break between episodes.

- How severe are the negative consequences caused by your depression? **Rate 0–10 _____, where:**

1 = **Mild:** I feel bad but there are no negative consequences.

5 = **Moderate:** My depression causes some serious problems in my life.

10 = **Severe:** My depression causes serious damage to my health, emotional well-being, and lifestyle.

Suicide Checklist

- I sometimes feel that life isn't worth living.

❏ Yes   ❏ No   ❏ Unsure

- I sometimes think I would be better off dead.

❏ Yes   ❏ No   ❏ Unsure

- I sometimes think about killing myself.

❏ Yes   ❏ No   ❏ Unsure

- I sometimes think about ways to kill myself.
  ☐ Yes   ☐ No   ☐ Unsure
- I have a plan to kill myself.
  ☐ Yes   ☐ No   ☐ Unsure
- I have recently tried to kill myself.
  ☐ Yes   ☐ No   ☐ Unsure
- I will probably try to kill myself some time in the future.
  ☐ Yes   ☐ No   ☐ Unsure

Note: If you answered "yes" or "unsure" to any of the last six questions, you may be seriously depressed and may need professional help immediately.

In the following table, you will see a checklist of symptoms that includes many of the symptoms typical for clinical depression. It's important to note, however, that only some of these symptoms are necessary for a diagnosis of depression. Some patients will be more comfortable with the depression rating instrument above, while others may benefit more from the following symptom list. Sometimes both can be useful.

Symptoms of Depression

- **A significantly depressed mood or general absence of mood:** You may sometimes feel yourself overly negative and down or at times emotionally cut off.
- **Inability to experience pleasure or feel interest in daily life:** Things that used to excite or interest you now hold no attraction at all. Sometimes it hardly seems worth getting up.
- **Inexplicable crying spells, sadness, and/or irritability:** You may find yourself crying for no reason or having a temper tantrum and lashing out without any provocation.
- **Insomnia (difficulty sleeping) or hyersomnia (oversleeping) nearly every day:** You either can't get to sleep or stay asleep and/or find yourself spending most of your time sleeping to the point of missing important events in your life.
- **A substantial change in appetite, eating patterns, or weight:** You find that you have no appetite and nothing sounds good so you just don't eat, or in an effort to feel better you discover that eating certain types of food seems to soothe you. You either lose or gain a significant amount of weight.

- **Fatigue or energy loss:** You seem to always be tired or don't seem to have enough energy to accomplish even simple tasks of daily living.
- **Diminished ability to concentrate:** You find that paying attention is very difficult. You may even find yourself reading the same page over and over or forgetting the plot of a movie you are watching.
- **Difficulty making decisions:** You can't seem to decide what to do even in simple areas that used to be easy for you. You tend to procrasitnate or put off having to decide.
- **Feelings of hopelessness or worthlessness:** At times you feel like your life is always going to be unbearable or you don't deserve to be happy or successful.
- **Inappropriate feelings of guilt or self-criticism:** You put yourself down for little things and feel bad about things that might not be your fault.
- **A lack of sexual drive:** You have lost your interest and passion for being a sexual being. It either seems like too much of a hassle or you just don't care anymore.
- **Suicidal thoughts, feelings, or behaviors:** You start having thoughts like "maybe I'd be better off dead," or "I feel that life isn't worth living." You may start thinking about ways you could kill yourself and even start developing a plan.

Treating Depression

One of the biggest problems in treating depression in people with chronic pain is missing the diagnosis. This occurs for two reasons: (1) The person in chronic pain often does not realize he or she is also suffering from a major depression, and (2) the healthcare provider is not looking for it. People living with chronic pain will often define their problem as strictly medical and related to the pain. Therefore, being alert to the possibility of depression and being willing to develop a treatment strategy becomes a crucial component of an effective pain management treatment plan.

There are currently a variety of highly effective interventions available for the treatment of depression. The majority of depressive conditions can be treated with either psychotherapy (especially cognitive behavioral therapy) or medication, but research studies have indicated that a combination of these interventions is usually the most effective form of treatment. There are also some types of depression that have a seasonal pattern where intensive Full Spectrum Lighting therapy is often effective in reducing symptoms. It should be emphasized that the majority of depressive conditions can be treated without hospitalization.

As you can see from the following chart, addictive disorders and depression are only two of the problematic coexisting disorders that this population faces. Unfortunately, it is beyond the scope of this book to go into the other disorders in the depth needed.

> Never underestimate the importance
> of using a team approach.

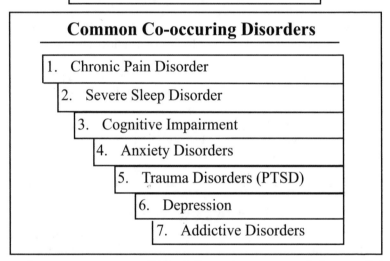

Common Co-occuring Disorders

1. Chronic Pain Disorder
2. Severe Sleep Disorder
3. Cognitive Impairment
4. Anxiety Disorders
5. Trauma Disorders (PTSD)
6. Depression
7. Addictive Disorders

As you can see, a multidisciplinary team approach is essential to gather accurate data in all five Axis areas. Teamwork also facilitates the implementation of the APM™ Core Clinical Exercises listed below.

• APM™ Core Clinical Exercise One: Understanding Your Pain

When diagnosing a pain disorder, it is essential to understand the difference between acute pain and chronic pain, especially when the pain may be managed with potentially addictive medication. It is also very important for the treatment professional to understand the biopsychosocial impact that a chronic pain condition has on a person.

In this section you will review the four parts of Exercise One in the *APM™ Workbook* that are designed to assist in gathering this information.

- **Exercise One, Part 1: Acute Pain versus Chronic Pain**

This exercise explains the difference between acute pain and chronic pain as well as describing the biopsychosocial effects of pain. The goal of this exercise is to increase patients' knowledge and understanding of pain and its effects in order to help them shift from the perception of themselves as a victim of pain, to one of being empowered to successfully manage their health.

As noted earlier, pain can be classified as either acute or chronic. Because the conditions are different, the treatment for acute pain is very different than the treatment for chronic pain. It is important to know the difference and be able to teach patients how to distinguish between the two.

Acute Pain

Acute pain tells the body that something has gone wrong or that damage to the system has occurred. The source of the pain can usually be easily identified, and typically, acute pain does not last very long. Acute pain is a symptom of an immediate underlying problem.

An example of acute pain is when someone touches a hot burner on the stove. Their first reaction is to pull away their hand. Contact with the heat will leave them with symptoms from minor redness to serious tissue damage, but in each case there is a predictable period of time for the burn to heal. There are also effective medical treatments that promote quick healing. Some other causes of acute pain include cuts and broken bones.

No matter what the source of acute pain, the result is to drive a person to search for relief. Once the problem is identified, it is standard and usually safe, unless the person has a history of substance abuse or dependency, to use analgesic and/or opiate medication for acute pain relief. If someone is in recovery for chemical dependency, an addiction medicine practitioner/specialist should be consulted before any opiate or other psychoactive medications are administered.

Acute Pain

- Gives an immediate signal to the brain
- Signals damage/dysfunction
- Is readily treatable
- Is of limited duration

Chronic Pain

Chronic pain is a condition that frequently fails to respond to standard medical interventions. In some cases there is no easily recognizable reason for the pain, or the original acute condition seems to be resolved but the pain signals keep firing. In addition, the pain has a duration of three to six months. The DSM-IV-TR criteria for a chronic condition is at least a six-month duration. In many cases chronic pain no longer serves a useful purpose; the pain system gets turned on and stays on well after the initial cause—or pain trigger—is resolved.

Dean and Jean present fairly typical examples of chronic pain conditions. Dean suffers from chronic knee pain. Although surgery and physical therapy have effectively treated the original injury, Dean's pain symptoms continued for years after his accident and also long after his surgery. Like many chronic pain patients, Dean was often told the pain was in his head. But to Dean the pain was very real and he wanted relief.

Chronic Pain

- Fails to respond to typical treatments
- Sometimes has no recognized source
- Lasts at least three to six months
- May no longer serve a useful purpose

Some other common chronic pain conditions include phantom limb pain, headaches, peripheral neuropathy, neck pain, and fibromyalgia. Chapter One presented a more in-depth explanation of pain that was designed to help you be more effective helping patients during this part of the APM™ treatment process.

Biopsychosocial Effects of Chronic Pain

People can generally receive effective medical care for acute pain; however, treatment for chronic pain can be a confusing process of misunderstanding as well as incorrect diagnoses and inadequate treatment plans.

When patients experience chronic pain and doctors are at a loss to define the exact nature of the problem, the patients might believe they are going crazy. Often treatment professionals will validate that belief, because they find no observable reason for the symptoms. However, chronic pain is real and often occurs for reasons that may not be identified easily. As explained earlier, chronic pain affects people physically, psychologically, socially, and spiritually—in body, mind, and spirit.

- Physically, chronic pain raises stress and drains physical energy.
- Psychologically, chronic pain affects the ability to think clearly, logically, and rationally, to manage feelings and emotions effectively.
- Socially, chronic pain affects the ability to use consistently responsible behaviors, thus affecting others.

Chronic Pain Affects a Person's	
Body	Thoughts
Emotions	Behaviors
Relationships	Pain Management

In addition, the way a person senses or experiences pain—its intensity and duration—will affect how well they are able to manage it. This goes back to our original discussion on pain versus suffering. Pain is an unpleasant signal telling us that something is wrong with our body. Suffering results from the meaning or interpretation we assign to the pain. Teaching patients more positive ways of thinking about their pain will lead to more effective pain management.

When a person has chronic pain, it is usually accepted that something is physically wrong with the body. The symptoms of pain can range from mildly irritating, to somewhat annoying or uncomfortable, to moderately distressing, to severely horrible, to the worst possible excruciating suffering!

113

While the patients are affected biologically, other areas are also impacted. Their thought processes are affected in several ways. Sometimes they might have difficulty thinking clearly or concentrating, which leads to being unable to solve problems that are normally easy for them. At times they may be unable to function very well in practically all areas of their life. Instead of thinking positively, they may repress certain thoughts and blank out, or indulge in self-defeating, negative, or depressive thinking.

Chronic pain can also lead to difficulty in managing emotions. Sometimes patients may be cut off from their emotions, become numb, and not know what they are feeling. At other times they may overreact to their emotions. The intensity of their feelings does not match the trigger situation. A third type of emotional dysfunction is when the patient experiences *artifact emotions*—feelings that do not seem to have a clear cause or trigger.

> Chronic pain often leads to depression.

As you saw earlier, many people with chronic pain also frequently become depressed. When their thinking is irrational or dysfunctional and they are mismanaging their feelings, they often have urges to indulge in self-defeating, impulsive, or compulsive behaviors to cope with their distress. This, in turn, affects their relationships with others. Some patients may become isolated and believe they can handle life without any help, or they may become overly dependent upon others to take care of them. This dysfunctional caretaking by others often enables the patient to continue ineffective behaviors that prolong their victim role.

The Biopsychosocial Sensation of Chronic Pain

Most chronic pain patients do not have the words they need to describe their pain. The first step in assessing and treating a chronic pain patient is to teach them the vocabulary they need in order to tell you about the type of pain they are experiencing. Remember that pain is a biopsychosocial experience. As a result you need to teach the patient to make a distinction between the physical sensation of pain, their psychological interpretation of the pain, and how they use their pain in relationships with other people.

- **Exercise One, Part 2-A: Identifying and Rating the Severity of Your Pain Symptoms**

This exercise has significantly evolved since the *APM™ Professional Guide* was first published in 1999. The original exercise was developed after reviewing several different pain assessment instruments (such as the McGuill Pain Assessment Questionnaire) that I have used with patients over the years. Through an active listening process I revised the original sixty-word list that most patients found useful in describing pain, to a list using fifty-four words. I call these words the *pain vocabulary.* This list has been revised and resequenced since the original work was published.

In order to help patients quickly find the words to describe their pain, the list is now organized into eighteen categories with three words in each category that progress from less severe to more severe pain and/or distress. This new list has an equal blend of physiological and psychological/emotional symptoms.

When someone has chronic pain, their sensation of pain and its effects vary. Exercise One, Part 2-A: Identifying and Rating the Severity of Your Pain Symptoms, in the *Addiction-Free Pain Management™ Workbook* offers an assessment tool to determine the level and intensity of both psychological and physiological symptoms. The physiological symptoms are the odd numbers, while the psychological emotional symptoms are the even-numbered groups.

Goals for Exercise One, Part 2-A
- Building a pain vocabulary
- Rating the severity of pain

The purpose of this exercise is twofold: to help patients build a vocabulary for talking about their pain and to explore their reactions to their pain in order to determine whether their condition is more physiological or psychological—pain versus suffering.

Look at the following chart describing the types of pain experienced by patients. Notice that the chart has three columns and eighteen rows. Each row contains three words that describe a certain symptom of pain. As you move from symptom one to symptom two and three, the words reflect an increasing intensity of that type of pain.

115

As patients read through each set of descriptions, they circle the word or words in each set that describe their sensations and write the appropriate number (on a scale of 1 to 10, with 1 meaning *low pain* and 10 meaning the *worst pain ever*) that best describes the intensity of their pain on a bad pain day.

This instrument shown below gives a chronic pain patient an increased vocabulary and insight to help them communicate accurately about their symptoms. This exercise along with Exercise One, Part 2-B, shows the patient there is a difference between physically-based symptoms and psychologically-based symptoms. At the same time it gives the clinician a deeper awareness of the issues that could influence successful treatment. It also provides additional assessment information. The patients are given the directions in the following table.

Instructions: When you have chronic pain, you are the only one that knows how it feels. Below are words (symptoms) that people with chronic pain can use to describe their pain. Not all will apply to you, but many of them will. The purpose of this worksheet is twofold: (1) to help you build a vocabulary for talking about your pain and (2) to rate the intensity or level of your pain. As you read through each three-word set, circle the **word(s)** and write in the **number** that best describes your pain on a **bad pain day**.

The Pain Vocabulary

Symptoms (Sensations of Chronic Pain)			Level
1. aching	throbbing	pulsing	
2. irritating	nagging	disturbing	
3. splitting	piercing	pounding	
4. dreadful	severe	awful	
5. irritated	sore	sensitive	
6. uncomfortable	troublesome	problematic	
7. burning	stinging	lacerating	
8. distressing	excruciating	agonizing	
9. tender	painful	hurtful	
10. worrisome	saddening	depressing	

11. inflamed	sharp	swollen
12. torturing	grueling	punishing
13. hot	radiating	spreading
14. annoying	upsetting	aggravating
15. tearing	wrenching	slashing
16. frightening	terrifying	dreadful
17. numbing	tingling	shooting
18. exhausting	fatiguing	debilitating
19. Is your pain more (A) permanent, constant, ceaseless; (B) fleeting, brief, momentary; or (C) combination of both?		
20. Why did you rate #19 that way?		

- **Exercise One, Part 2-B:**
  Exploring Biological versus Psychological Pain Symptoms

Ascending and Descending Pain Signals

Once the patients have completed Exercise One, Part 2-A, they need to immediately go to Exercise One, Part 2-B to learn about the physiological versus psychological/emotional components of their pain. The following table lists the directions for completing that exercise.

Ascending pain signals, coming from the point of injury to the brain, and *descending* nerve pathways, signals from the brain to the point of injury, will influence or modify the effects of pain on your body.

Some of these ascending signals simply report the presence of pain (I hurt or I don't hurt). Other signals report the intensity of the pain (It hurts a little or it hurts a lot). Still other pain signals report the location of the pain (My stomach hurts) or whether the pain is associated with an internal or external injury (My stomach hurts deep in my gut, or the skin on my stomach hurts). Other pain signals report the type of pain (It burns or it throbs).

All of these different pain signals are transmitted into the spinal cord through nerve pathways to the hypothalamus section of the brain. There the brain transmits the pain signal information to other specialized pain neurons, which in turn sends the information (descending signals) to different areas in the brain. One area that gets the message is your limbic system—this is the emotional center of the brain. It leads to a feeling or emotional response. Another signal goes to your frontal lobes—this is the cognition/thinking center of the brain. It leads to thoughts or judgments about your pain, including *anticipatory pain*.

Once the physical pain system is activated, the anticipatory pain reaction can actually make pain symptoms worse. Whenever you feel the pain, you *interpret it* in a way that makes it worse. You *start thinking* about the pain in a way that makes it worse. You *tell yourself* that the pain is "awful and terrible," and think, "I can't handle the pain." You *convince yourself*, "It's hopeless, I'll always hurt, and there's nothing that I can do about it."

Below are the same pain symptoms you identified and rated earlier in the previous exercise—Identifying and Rating the Severity of Your Pain Symptoms—but in a slightly different format. You will notice that the *odd-numbered* items from the worksheet are now in the left-hand (ascending) column, while the *even-numbered* items are in the right-hand (descending) column. This is where anticipatory pain is created.

Next you will have an opportunity to identify your ascending and descending pain signals. Take a few minutes to transpose the circled symptoms and numeric ratings from the previous exercise to the exercise on the next page. Then add up the total of the numbered ratings for each column. Remember that it really doesn't matter how you score as long as you are willing to use this as a self-monitoring system to help you better manage your pain.

Ascending/Biological Pain Signals	Descending/Psychological Pain Signals
1. aching, throbbing, pulsing Rating =	2. irritating, nagging, disturbing Rating =
3. splitting, piercing, pounding Rating =	4. dreadful, severe, awful Rating =
5. irritated, sore, sensitive Rating =	6. uncomfortable, troublesome, problematic Rating =
7. burning, stinging, lacerating Rating =	8. distressing, excruciating, agonizing Rating =
9. tender, painful, hurtful Rating =	10. worrisome, saddening, depressing Rating =
11. inflamed, sharp, swollen Rating =	12. torturing, grueling, punishing Rating =
13. hot, radiating, spreading Rating =	14. annoying, upsetting, aggravating Rating =
15. tearing, wrenching, slashing Rating =	16. frightening, terrifying, dreadful Rating =
17. numbing, tingling, shooting Rating =	18. exhausting, fatiguing, debilitating Rating =
Total Ascending = _____	**Total Descending** = _____

> Now let's look at the results of Jean and Dean's
> exercise to see what can be learned.

Let's start by looking at how Dean and Jean completed Exercise One, Part 2-A: Identifying and Rating the Severity of Your Pain Symptoms and how they transposed their symptoms onto the worksheet below. The symptoms they circled are shown in the table below in **bold/underlined** and the level (or rating) is at the end of each row.

Dean's Pain Symptoms on a Bad Pain Day

Ascending Symptoms	Rating	Descending Symptoms	Rating
1. **aching**, throbbing, pulsing	7	2. irritating, **nagging**, **disturbing**	8
3. splitting, **piercing**, pounding	6	4. dreadful, **severe**, **awful**	10
5. **irritated**, sore, sensitive	7	6. **uncomfortable**, **troublesome**, problematic	9
7. **burning**, stinging, **lacerating**	6	8. **distressing**, excruciating, **agonizing**	9
9. **tender**, **painful**, hurtful	7	10. **worrisome**, **saddening**, **depressing**	10
11. **inflamed**, **sharp**, swollen	7	12. torturing, grueling, **punishing**	10
13. **hot**, radiating, **spreading**	6	14. **annoying**, upsetting, **aggravating**	10
15. tearing, wrenching, **slashing**	7	16. **frightening**, terrifying, **dreadful**	10
17. numbing, tingling, **shooting**	7	18. **exhausting**, **fatiguing**, debilitating	10
Total Ascending = **60**		**Total Descending** = **86**	

Jean's Pain Symptoms on a Bad Pain Day

Ascending Symptoms	Rating	Descending Symptoms	Rating
1. aching, **throbbing**, pulsing	10	2. **irritating**, nagging, **disturbing**	10
3. splitting, **piercing**, pounding	10	4. **dreadful**, **severe**, **awful**	10
5. irritated, **sore**, **sensitive**	8	6. uncomfortable, **troublesome**, **problematic**	10
7. **burning**, **stinging**, lacerating	6	8. **distressing**, **excruciating**, **agonizing**	10
9. tender, **painful**, **hurtful**	8	10. **worrisome**, **saddening**, **depressing**	10
11. **inflamed**, sharp, **swollen**	6	12. **torturing**, grueling, **punishing**	10
13. **hot**, radiating, spreading	6	14. annoying, **upsetting**, **aggravating**	10
15. tearing, wrenching, **slashing**	7	16. **frightening**, **terrifying**, **dreadful**	10
17. **numbing**, **tingling**, shooting	7	18. **exhausting**, fatiguing, **debilitating**	10
Total Ascending = __68__		**Total Descending** = __90__	

Scoring the Ascending and Descending Pain Signals Exercise

After the patients are finished transposing the numbers from the first instrument to the one above, they are given more information about what their answers mean. This is where it is important to normalize that patients will experience both physiological as well as psychological/emotional symptoms. After being given this information, patients are asked to commit to learning more. Please see the remainder of the Ascending/Descending exercise reproduced in the table below.

You will get a chance to look at this exercise further on the following pages, especially when developing your *Pain Flare-Up Plan*. It is very important to remember that when you have pain, there are three components to that pain: (1) biological; (2) psychological/emotional; and (3) social/cultural. All three components need to be treated, but the treatment plan for each differs. An effective medication management plan coupled with nonpharmacological interventions is the best approach for the biological pain symptoms.

However, using medication for the psychological/emotional symptoms is like having an infected cut on your hand and the only thing you do for it is to find a color-coordinated bandage and slap it on. Using medication for the psychological/emotional symptoms puts you at risk for experiencing negative side effects from your medication, including potential addiction problems. The good news is there are ways you can learn to identify and cope with your psychological/emotional symptoms. It is also important to identify any social and/or cultural beliefs/biases that could potentially sabotage an effective pain management plan. Are you willing to make a commitment to learn more effective pain management tools?

❐ Yes   ❐ No   ❐ Unsure
Please explain:

What Do Dean and Jean's Answers Mean?

Several points stand out when reviewing Dean's completed exercise. Dean scored significantly higher in the *descending* area, which is not uncommon for someone living with chronic pain and a coexisting addictive disorder. Dean's first reaction was that he was being manipulated and tricked. This also is a common reaction, especially for patients who have trust issues. Dean eventually learned to use this ascending/descending process as a part of his daily pain journal work.

> Psychological/emotional pain is real!
> It also needs appropriate interventions.

At this point in the *APM™ Workbook* process it is important to go into more depth about the ascending versus descending pain symptoms and normalize the fact that no matter which it is—pain is pain and it needs appropriate intervention. Dean was very excited to hear he could learn simple-to-implement, nonmedication ways to help him cope with his descending pain symptoms. His interest increased as I told him he would be developing a nonpharmacological pain flare-up plan in a following exercise.

Now let's review Jean's answers for the same exercise. As with Dean, several points stand out when looking through Jean's completed exercise, including the fact that she scored higher in the descending area. The first important observation about Jean's descending symptoms is that she scored them **all** at a level 10. There are several reasons this happens; the most important is that patients may have never been taught how to understand and complete a pain rating scale. Like Jean you will get a chance to learn more about how to accurately use both stress and pain scales in Exercise One, Part 4: Stress and Chronic Pain.

Another reason why many patients, including Jean, score the descending symptoms so high is they think that no one would help them if they didn't make their problem seem serious enough. In fact, that has proven to be true in many research studies on pain behaviors impacting pain interventions by healthcare providers. Later in treatment Jean also disclosed that rating her pain levels high was her justification for getting more, and taking more, pain medication; once she convinced herself of that, it was much easier to convince her doctor. When Jean completed this exercise and saw her scores and what they meant, she was shocked. After processing this exercise with her she became much more hopeful and eager to continue the APM™ process, especially when, like Dean, she looked ahead to the pain flare-up plan exercise.

The next stage of the work was to help Jean and Dean to begin noticing how their thinking, emotions, and behaviors changed when they were experiencing a bad pain day. This next exercise is primarily focused on the problem, and in Exercise Seven you will see how Dean and Jean learned to manage similar problematic thoughts, emotions, and behaviors and move into the solution.

- **Exercise One, Part 3: Exploring Your TFUARs on a Bad Pain Day**

> The primary goal of *"Exploring Your TFUARs"* is to see how irrational thinking leads to emotional and social distress.

The acronym TFUAR means:

T = Thoughts, F = Feelings, U = Urges, A = Actions, R = Reactions

This exercise is designed to explore addictive or irrational thinking (thinking errors) that occur as a result of a chronic pain condition. That type of thinking often leads to uncomfortable emotions that trigger self-defeating urges, usually followed by self-destructive behaviors. The following table lists the questions asked in this *APM™ Workbook* exercise. Some patients will need coaching in order to come up with answers in all the TFUAR categories. Sometimes it is helpful to do imagery exercises and ask people to reexperience a bad pain day and tell it like a story. This technique is explained in-depth in the High-Risk Situation Mapping Exercise later in the book.

Exploring Your TFUARs Exercise
When you experience a bad pain day, your TFUARs (thinking, feelings, urges, actions, and reactions of others) often change. The purpose of this exercise is to explore your personal accounts in each of the above TFUAR areas when you experience pain on a bad pain day. You will do more with this TFUAR process later in the book.
Thinking: Prolonged exposure to chronic pain leads to irrational thinking (thinking errors) and self-defeating decision making. List below three thinking problems that you've experienced as a result of your pain.
Feelings: Use the Feelings Chart below to describe how you feel when you're experiencing chronic pain at its worst, and how intense each feeling is on a scale of 0 (lowest intensity) to 10 (highest intensity).

The Feelings Checklist Chart			
Strong	or	Weak	How strong is the feeling? (0–10) _____
Safe	or	Threatened	How strong is the feeling? (0–10) _____
Angry	or	Caring	How strong is the feeling? (0–10) _____
Fulfilled	or	Frustrated	How strong is the feeling? (0–10) _____

Happy	or	Sad	How strong is the feeling? (0–10) _____
Connected	or	Lonely	How strong is the feeling? (0–10) _____
Proud	or	Ashamed/Guilty	How strong is the feeling? (0–10) _____
Peaceful	or	Agitated	How strong is the feeling? (0–10) _____

Urges:	What do you have an urge (or impulse) to do when you're experiencing chronic pain at its worst?
Actions:	What do you usually do when you're experiencing chronic pain at its worst?
Reactions:	When you are experiencing chronic pain at its worst, how do other people usually react?
How do those reactions by other people affect your stress and/or pain levels?	

The purpose of this exercise is twofold. First, it gives clinicians insight into their patients' psychological (cognition and affect), behavioral, and social patterns. Second, it gives patients a new way of looking at how their pain experiences often have a number of undesirable biopsychosocial consequences.

For example, Dean identified his three irrational thinking patterns: (1) I don't deserve this; (2) I have to do whatever it takes to stop this; and (3) I won't use meds next time, but this time I really need help. Dean tends to react in a top-dog (power) fashion. Jean, on the other hand, came up with three underdog (victim) statements: (1) I'm such a bad mother. (2) Why won't they let me get relief? (3) This is too much to deal with.

Both Jean and Dean identified similar feelings: weak, angry, sad, lonely, threatened, and frustrated. Jean rated weak at level 10 while Dean rated it level 5. Jean rated sad at a level 8 and Dean rated it 4. Both rated angry and frustrated at a level 10, and Jean rated ashamed at level 10. Dean did not rate either proud or ashamed— Dean later admitted he was in denial about his shame. Both also rated agitated at a level 10.

Both Jean and Dean had an urge to use inappropriate pain medication. Dean did often overuse his pain medication on a bad pain day, and if there was not enough available, he would find other ways to distract himself. Recently he started having urges to drink again. Jean tended to cry or try to go to sleep to escape if she did not have enough pain medication.

Both Jean and Dean tended to isolate. Dean hid his pain with a tough-guy facade, and Jean reported she was feeling too much shame and guilt to reach out. The result was that they closed themselves off from any support networks. Isolation is a common tendency for a chronic pain patient; this problem becomes much worse if they also have a coexisting addictive disorder.

- **Exercise One, Part 4: Stress and Chronic Pain**

> **Primary Goal:**
> To show patients the connection between stress and pain

The *TFUAR* exercise is followed by the Stress and Chronic Pain scales exercise in the following table. This exercise will be discussed in greater detail in a later chapter.

It is important to know about the connection between stress levels and your pain symptoms, as well as understanding that stress management can also decrease your suffering. Physically, chronic pain raises your stress level and drains physical energy, while psychologically if affects your ability to think clearly, logically, and rationally, as well as to effectively manage your feelings or emotions. Remember that in most cases if you can learn to lower your stress levels, you will also experience a decrease in your perception of pain.

When you are more aware of your stress levels, you can then take action to reduce your stress, which in turn leads to a decrease in your pain symptoms. One effective stress management strategy is exercise. In addition to lowering your stress levels, regular exercise can also be an important part of your pain management program. It is also important to reduce—or even eliminate—nicotine, caffeine, and sugar, and implement a healthy eating plan. Other stress management tools could include focused breathing and relaxation exercises, meditation, Yoga, Tai Chi, soothing music, being in nature, soaking in a hot bath (or Jacuzzi), etc.

Of course before you learn to manage your stress, you need to be familiar with ways to assess your level of stress. It is important to learn how to accurately self-assess your levels of stress, then learn how to develop some simple but effective stress management tools. I like to use the Gorski-CENAPS® *Stress Thermometer* concept for stress identification. This concept proposes that there are ten levels of stress. When you get to the upper moderate to severe levels of stress (6–10 range), your thinking, emotions, and behavior are impacted. Below are examples of stress scales and the stress thermomether for you to review.

General Stress Levels and the Stress Thermometer

General Stress Levels

Low Stress Level (stress score: 1–3)

    1 Very relaxed; vacation mode

    2 Stress is managed well; no discomfort

    3 No Notable distress or dysfunction

Moderate Stress Levels (stress score: 4–6)

    4 Higher stress levels: normal operating level, no distress

    5 Stress managed poorly at times; some discomfort but no distress

    6 Some notable distress but minimal dysfunction

Severe Stress Levels (stress score: 7–10)

    7 Very high stress levels

    8 Stress is usually managed poorly

    9 Stress causes notable distress and dysfunction

Score 7	=	**I Space Out**
Score 8	=	**I Get Defensive**
Score 9	=	**I Overreact**
Score 10	=	**I Can't Function (or run away)**

The Stress Thermometer		
Trauma Reaction	10	Loss of Control
	9	Overreact
Stress Reaction	8	Get Driven/Defensive
	7	Space Out
	6	Free Flow with Effort
Functional Stress	5	Free Flow with No Effort
	4	Focused and Active
	3	Relaxed—Focused
Relaxation	2	Relaxed—Not Focused
	1	Relaxed—Nearly Asleep

Often with chronic pain, as stress levels go up, so does the level of your pain. Think of a time when you were experiencing very low levels of pain and for some reason your stress levels went up. What happened to your level of pain? Most likely it also increased.

Periodically throughout this workbook you should monitor both your level of stress and your level of pain. When asked to describe your pain or stress levels, use the stress scale above and the pain scale that follows, using the 1- to 10-point rating system. You also want to be aware of whether your pain is more physiological (biological) or psychological/emotional. Come up with a personalized short descriptor of each of the ten levels of pain to make the following pain scale work the best for you. For example, what words would describe your level 7 pain?

Looking at Two Pain Scales

1	2	3	4	5	6	7	8	9	10

Mild or No Pain	Uncomfortable Pain	Distressing Pain	Terrible Pain	Agonizing Pain

The second way to look at describing your pain level is by using a brief ten-point scale with short descriptors like the following one. As you review this ten-point scale, think how you would describe each of the ten levels in your own words. The important thing is for you to learn how to communicate your levels of pain accurately to your healthcare provider.

Level 1 = My pain is barely noticeable.

Level 2 = My pain is noticeable with no distress.

Level 3 = My pain is becoming disturbing but I have no distress.

Level 4 = My pain is causing me some distress but I have no coping problems.

Level 5 = My pain is causing me distress and I have some coping problems.

Level 6 = My pain is causing me distress and I have significant coping problems.

Level 7 = My pain is starting to interfere with my ability to function.

Level 8 = My pain is causing moderate interference with my ability to function.

Level 9 = My pain is causing severe interference with my ability to function.

Level 10 = I'm unable to function at all because of my pain.

Using the above scales, answer the following:
1. On my best days I would rate my pain at level _____ and my stress would be at level _____.
2. On an average day I would rate my pain at level _____ and my stress would be at level _____.
3. On my worst days I would rate my pain at level _____ and my stress would be at level _____.

Many people find there is a definite correlation between their stress and their level of pain. That is why a good stress management plan is crucial for someone living with chronic pain. It is even more important if you are also in recovery from an addictive disorder, because stress turns on or exacerbates something called Protracted or Post Acute Withdrawal.

As you are looking at the exercise—*Looking at Two Pain Scales*—think back to how you completed your *Identifying and Rating the Severity of Your Pain Symptoms* exercise. After looking at this pain level information, would you rate your symptoms the same way? Many people find they overrated the levels of their pain. However, some people find they actually underrated their symptoms the first time.

Patients are asked to use these charts to rate their pain and stress on their best days, on an average day, and on their worst pain day. The goal of this exercise is to help patients see that pain and stress are connected and good stress management can often reduce the intensity of pain.

Some patients have difficulty in accurately rating and communicating the type and levels of their pain. Some patients can benefit from using the pain scale in the exercise above, but others may need more help. One way is to have them give a verbal description of each of the 1–10 levels of pain starting at level one. Jean was able to do this quite easily, but Dean needed more help. So he was given the APM™ Expanded Pain Scale shown in the following table.

The APM™ Expanded Pain Scale

0	=	The absence of any pain signals
1–3	=	When I have pain at this level, my pain is a nuisance but I can almost always function normally without any extra effort. At these levels I might describe my pain as mildly troubling but no big deal. Most of the time I might not even notice that I'm in pain.
4–6	=	When I experience this level of pain, at times I can function normally with extra effort and at other times I struggle. At this level I might describe my pain as frustrating or even aggravating. When my pain gets to level six, it starts to feel like a very big deal, and I'm always conscious of being in pain.
7–10	=	When I reach this level of pain, most of the time I can't function normally even with medication and extra effort. At this level I'm truly "suffering" and might describe my pain as awful, horrible, or unbearable. When my pain gets to the 9–10 levels, I sometimes panic and mistakenly believe that it will never get better.

Both Jean and Dean were able to quickly see the connection between their stress and pain levels, and they used these scales throughout the remainder of their treatment. In many instances they both were able to report using stress identification and management to reduce their pain symptoms.

Once patients are able to describe their pain symptoms and understand the biopsychosocial effects, the next task is to explore their use of pain medication. Prescription medication and other drugs (including alcohol) change how the brain and nervous system work. These substances may slow it down, speed it up, block it out, change, or "blow up" (amplify) the messages and feelings that are sent out by the brain. These drug effects make people feel different for a little while, but they don't actually change anything in the real world. They usually only mask the chronic pain and change how people think, feel, and act. But the medication does not usually make their life any better—in fact, their life often gets worse.

In the next chapter you will see how Jean and Dean completed Exercise Two from the *APM™ Workbook*. In it you will learn the importance of educating patients about the biopsychosocial effects of their medication and how the APM™ approach teaches them to make appropriate decisions regarding the use of their medication.

- **Call to Action for the Fourth Chapter**

It is time to summarize what you learned so far now that you have come to the end of the fourth chapter. Please answer the questions below.

1. What is the most important thing you have learned about yourself and your ability to help addicted pain patients as a result of completing Chapter Four?

2. What are you willing to commit to do differently as a result of what you have learned by completing this chapter?

3. What obstacles might get in the way of making these changes? What can you do to overcome these roadblocks?

**Take time to pause and reflect, then
go to the next page to review Chapter Five.**

Chapter Five

Effects of Prescription and/or Other Drugs

• Pain Relief versus Euphoria

Some patients with chronic pain who use addictive medication for pain management never experience negative consequences. So why do other patients develop an addictive disorder? The answer to this often depends upon various factors, such as genetics, coexisting disorders, and environmental dynamics. For further comprehension it is also important to have an expanded understanding of addiction. In Chapter One you learned about the addictive disorder process that occurs and were introduced to the following chart.

1.	Euphoria	6.	Inability to Abstain
2.	Craving	7.	Addiction-Centered Lifestyle
3.	Tolerance	8.	Addictive Lifestyle Losses
4.	Loss of Control	9.	Continued Use Despite Problems
5.	Withdrawal	10.	Substance-Induced Organic Mental Disorders

As you saw earlier, Dean was finally able to break through his denial and admit that he often used his pain medication for its *euphoric effects*. This is a common realization for many chronic pain patients. It is important to explore this further, using the information from the *Biopsychosocial Model of Alcoholism and Drug Addiction* (Gorski, 1999).

Understanding Euphoria

So why is there a transition that chronic pain patients make when they go from using the pain medication for pain relief to using it either for emotional coping or perhaps for its euphoric effects? This question can be answered, in part, by understanding the relationship of brain reward mechanisms and the behavior of using psychoactive medication, or alcohol and other drugs.

The brain reward mechanism demonstrates that the tendency toward drug-seeking behavior is strongly linked to progressive alterations in the function of the brain, and in late stages to the development of structural damage to the brain and other organ systems.

The NIAAA (National Institute on Alcohol Abuse and Alcoholism) research clearly shows there are biomedical processes that occur within the brain that reinforce the regular and heavy use of psychoactive chemicals.

These *biomedical brain reinforcement processes* are different from the classic withdrawal syndrome. The following is a summary of this research reported in the Alcohol Alert from NIAAA for July of 1996. It continues to be relevant.

The Biomedical Brain Reinforcement Process

- People will tend to repeat an action that brings pleasure or reward. The pleasure or reward provided by that action is called *positive reinforcement* or *euphoria*.

- Certain behaviors, especially those associated with survival needs, are linked to biochemical processes within the brain that cause powerful *biological reinforcement* for these behaviors.

- This biological reinforcement is related to the release of specific brain chemicals when the behavior is performed. These brain chemicals produce a sense of pleasure or reward.

- Alcohol and Other Drugs of Abuse (AODs), including medications, produce chemicals that are surrogates of the naturally occurring brain chemicals that produce biological reinforcement.

- As a result the use of AODs causes a rewarding mental state (euphoria) that positively reinforces the initial use of AODs. This rewarding mental state is defined as euphoria. (Euphoria is a state that is separate and distinct from the symptoms of intoxication.)

- As a result, individuals who receive positive reinforcement for AOD use, because of the production of these brain chemicals, are more likely to engage in drug-seeking behavior and to use drugs regularly and heavily.

- The biochemical reinforcement that results from alcohol and drug use is more powerful and persistently reinforcing than the biomedical reinforcement provided by other survival-related actions.

- This perception that alcohol and drug use is more important than meeting other survivaly needs results in *drug-seeking behavior*.

- After drug-seeking behavior has been established, the brain undergoes certain adaptive changes to continue functioning despite the presence of the chemicals. This adaptation is called *tolerance*.

- This low-grade, abstinence-based brain dysfunction is distinct and different from the traditional acute withdrawal symptoms.

- This low-grade, abstinence-based brain dysfunction is marked by feelings of discomfort, cravings, and difficulty finding gratification from other behaviors.

- This creates a desire to avoid the unpleasant sensations that occur in abstinence. This desire to avoid painful stimuli is called *negative reinforcement*.

- People who experience biological reinforcement (both positive and negative) are more likely to use drugs regularly and heavily.

- People who use drugs regularly and heavily are more likely to develop

  –physical dependence syndromes marked by tolerance and classic withdrawal symptoms and

  –biomedical complications resulting from alcohol and drug use.

- There is evidence that people who are genetically and prenatally exposed to addiction may have pathological brain reward mechanisms.

- This pathological brain reward mechanism is marked by a below average release of packets of brain reward chemicals when not using the drug of choice.

  –When the drug of choice is used, the brain releases abnormally large amounts of brain reward chemicals.

  –When sober, the person experiences a sense of decreased wellbeing that is marked by a low grade agitated depression and *anhedonia*—the ability to experience pleasure.

  –This feeling creates a craving for something, anything that will relieve the feeling.

- When the person finds the drug of choice that releases large amounts of brain reward chemicals, the person experiences a powerful sense of pleasure or euphoria. The experience feels so good the patient begins seeking that experience.

> This biomedical condition leads to psychological and social reinforcement.

Psychological Reinforcement

The mind is capable of formulating thoughts that produce strong, positive biological reinforcement. These thoughts often take the form of positive judgments about behavior and reflect in self-talk, such as "Doing this is good for me!"

Positive judgments about behavior can be reinforcing of and by themselves because they are capable of activating the release of the biologically reinforcing brain chemicals. When this occurs, the positive judgment is said to *trigger* the state of reinforcement.

> Psychological Reinforcement = Gratification

When the biologically reinforcing brain chemicals are automatically released in response to a behavior, the person feels pleasure and is more likely to judge the behavior as positive, which stimulates the release of more reinforcing brain chemicals. When this occurs, the judgment a person makes is said to *enhance* the state of reinforcement.

Social Reinforcement

Social reinforcement occurs when the behavior of others or the response of the environment is judged to be positive. These positive judgments about how people and the environment respond to us can trigger or enhance biological reinforcement.

> Social Reinforcement = Reward

For chronic pain patients who have addictive disorders and may need to use APM™ Medication Management Components, special precautions must be taken. It is important to know how to determine whether or not the medication is being used appropriately.

That is why the *Pain Medication Recovery and Relapse Indicators* chart shown below was developed. Using this checklist, combined with Exercise Two from the *Addiction-Free Pain Management™ Workbook*, gives patients and healthcare providers a better chance of avoiding potential problems.

Pain Medication Recovery and Relapse Indicators

Recovery Indicators	Relapse Indicators
1. Patient is using medication as prescribed and in accordance with their *Medication Management Treatment Plan*.	1. Patient is not using medication as prescribed, or is not in accordance with their *Medication Management Treatment Plan*.
2. Patient is using pain medication only for its analgesic pain relief.	2. Patient is using pain medication for its euphoric effects and/or its emotional management properties.
3. Patient is not experiencing obsession for or intrusive thoughts about the medication.	3. Patient is experiencing obsession for and/or intrusive thoughts about the medication.
4. Patient is not experiencing compulsion to use the medication.	4. Patient is experiencing compulsion to use the medication.
5. Patient is not experiencing a craving to use the medication.	5. Patient is experiencing a craving to use the medication.
6. Patient is not experiencing a loss of control of the medication.	6. Patient is experiencing a loss of control of the medication.
7. Patient is not experiencing intoxication from using the medication.	7. Patient is experiencing intoxication from using the medication.
8. Patient is not experiencing negative biological consequences from using the medication.	8. Patient is experiencing negative biological consequences from using the medication.
9. Patient is not experiencing any secondary psychological related problems due to using the medication.	9. Patient is experiencing secondary psychological related problems due to using the medication.
10. Patient is not experiencing a pain rebound effect from using the medication.	10. Patient is experiencing a pain rebound effect from using the medication.

Expectations versus Reality

- **Exercise Two, Part 1: Effects of Prescription and/or Other Drugs**

In Exercise Two, Part 1: "What you Wanted and What you Got" exercise, patients are asked to list the type(s), amount(s), and frequency of the medication(s) they are currently using (or have used) to manage their pain. Alcohol needs to be included, because many people with chronic pain often use alcohol to help manage their pain.

Patients then explore what they wanted the drugs to do, the effects the drugs actually produced that made them believe they were getting what they wanted, and finally, what they learned from completing the exercise.

At this point it would be extremely beneficial to consult with the patient's primary physician. If that doctor is not certified in addiction medicine, someone with that training should also be consulted. See the following table to review this exercise.

Prescription medication and other drugs (including alcohol) change how the brain and nervous system work. They slow down, speed up, block out, change, or "blow up" the messages and feelings that your brain sends out. These drug effects make you feel different for a little while, but they don't actually change anything in the real world. They mask your chronic pain and change how you think, feel, and act, but usually they don't make your life any better—in fact, they make life much worse.

In the following exercises you will be asked to list the type, amount, and frequency of the medication you are currently using (or have used during the past year) to manage your pain. Alcohol needs to be included because many people with chronic pain often use alcohol to help manage their pain. Some people also use some of the illicit drugs, e.g., marijuana, methamphetamine. If you use those chemicals, list them as well. You will then explore what you wanted the drugs to do, the effects the drugs produced that made you believe you were getting what you wanted, and what you learned as a result of completing this exercise.

Part 1-A: What You Used and How Well It Worked

In this section list each drug you used for pain management (including alcohol or other nonprescribed drugs), how much you used, how often you used it, how long the effects lasted, and how much relief you received. Rate the amount of relief on a 1 to 10 scale, with 1 being very minimal and 10 being total relief.

Part 1-B: What You Wanted Your Medication to Do

Please answer each of the following questions as fully and honestly as you can.

---

1. What are the three most important things you wanted your pain medication to do for you?

2. Could you do these things for yourself without using pain medication?

   ☐ Yes   ☐ No   ☐ Unsure   Please explain:

3. What are the three most important things you wanted the pain medication to help you cope with or escape from?

4. Can you cope with or escape from these things without using pain medication?

   ☐ Yes   ☐ No   ☐ Unsure   Please explain:

5. Looking back on it now, do you think that the pain medication did for you what you wanted it to do?

   ☐ Yes   ☐ No   ☐ Unsure   Please explain:

Part 1-C: What You Learned

6. List below the three most important things you have learned as a result of completing this exercise.

7. What are you willing to do differently as a result of what you learned?

Remember—Teamwork Is a Must!

The second part of Exercise Two explores some of the most common side effects and problems experienced from using pain medication. In some instances prescription medication and other drugs (including alcohol) have been beneficial, in the short run, for pain management. However, these chemicals, psychoactive interventions, often have serious physical side effects and/or lead to psychological and social problems.

- **Exercise Two, Part 2: Side Effects and Problems**

Some of the most common side effects people experience from their pain medication are listed below. Patients are asked to indicate how each of these applies to them, rating the degree of impact by circling the appropriate number (on a scale of 1 to 10, with 1 being not a problem to 10 being extremely problematic).

Effects of Substances Exercise

1. Increased tolerance (needing more of the drug)
2. Nausea and/or vomiting
3. Feeling sleepy, fatigued, or drowsy
4. Becoming short-tempered (easily angered)
5. Impaired liver functions
6. Abdominal pain or cramping
7. Feeling down or depressed
8. Thoughts of suicide
9. Decreased sexuality or libido
10. Increased anxiety
11. Increased family or relationship problems
12. Euphoria—feeling high (intoxicated)
13. Becoming confused or disoriented
14. Blurred and/or double vision
15. Stomach pain and/or ulcers
16. Being dependent/addicted
17. Urine retention
18. Diarrhea
19. Decreased job performance
20. Difficulty having fun or experiencing pleasure

Jean's Answers to the Effects of Substances Exercise

Effects of Substances

	Level
1. Increased tolerance (needing more of the drug)	9
2. Nausea and/or vomiting	2
3. Feeling sleepy, fatigued, or drowsy	4
4. Becoming short-tempered (easily angered)	8
5. Impaired liver functions	2
6. Abdominal pain or cramping	4
7. Feeling down or depressed	8

8. Thoughts of suicide	3
9. Decreased sexuality or libido	9
10. Increased anxiety	10
11. Increased family or relationship problems	8
12. Euphoria—feeling high (intoxicated)	8
13. Becoming confused or disoriented	8
14. Blurred and/or double vision	1
15. Stomach pain and/or ulcers	4
16. Being dependent/addicted	10
17. Urine retention	1
18. Diarrhea	1
19. Decreased job performance	8
20. Difficulty having fun or experiencing pleasure	9

On her first attempt to complete this exercise, Jean had greatly underrated many of the symptoms. As she processed the results during session, she began to see how much she minimized the negative consequences and only focused on the benefits of the medication.

Jean's second attempt was much more honest and showed an increase in most of the categories (listed above). This exercise also opened up the discussion about other ways her use of pain medication was negatively impacting her life, as well as being problematic for her family and friends.

Now let's look at how Dean completed this exercise.

Dean's Answers to the Effects of Substances Exercise

Effects of Substances	Level
1. Increased tolerance (needing more of the drug)	8
2. Nausea and/or vomiting	2
3. Feeling sleepy, fatigued, or drowsy	3
4. Becoming short-tempered (easily angered)	9
5. Impaired liver functions	2
6. Abdominal pain or cramping	2

7.	Feeling down or depressed	10
8.	Thoughts of suicide	4
9.	Decreased sexuality or libido	10
10.	Increased anxiety	10
11.	Increased family or relationship problems	10
12.	Euphoria—feeling high (intoxicated)	8
13.	Becoming confused or disoriented	9
14.	Blurred and/or double vision	1
15.	Stomach pain and/or ulcers	3
16.	Being dependent/addicted	10
17.	Urine retention	2
18.	Diarrhea	2
19.	Decreased job performance	10
20.	Difficulty having fun or experiencing pleasure	10

Dean was honest with his evaluation and reported that it was painful for him to see all these negative side effects listed on paper. He also noted that this pain had never stopped him from using before, but now he wanted to learn how to use this information to increase his positive self-talk. Again it was the *processing* of the exercise that had the most impact—not just filling out the forms.

> It is very important to uncover the patient's beliefs about pain, as well as the benefits and disadvantages of taking the pain medication.

The next step in the assessment process is determining the person's beliefs about pain medication, their earliest experiences around pain and medication, and their perceived benefits and disadvantages of using pain medication.

• Exercise Three: Decision Making about Pain Medication

Exercise Three in the *Addiction-Free Pain Management*™ *Workbook* is a series of four decision-making exercises, which are designed to assist the chemical dependency/abuse assessment process. Part 1 explores personal beliefs about pain and medication.

Exercise Three, Part 1:
Your Personal Beliefs about Pain and Medication

Often the decision to use pain medication has been made because a doctor prescribed it, usually after a very brief consultation with the patient. Many doctors have minimal training in addictive disorders and may not be aware of the risks for some patients. On the other hand, some people mislead their doctors (intentionally or unintentionally) by not giving them an accurate picture of their past history with alcohol or other drug problems. Other factors in medication decision making center on a person's response to and beliefs about pain.

Prerequisites of APM™ Recovery

- Honest self-evaluation
- Accurate self-monitoring
- Healthy self-changing behaviors

The overall purpose of this exercise is for patients to explore how they make decisions so they can begin to make accurate, honest, and healthy choices about pain management and pain medication.

Patients are asked to think back to the very first time they took any medication (including alcohol) for pain relief and write about it like a story with a beginning, middle, and end. They are told to make sure to include: their age at the time, what they were doing, who they were with, what happened, what thoughts they had about their pain, how they were affected or what feelings were produced by the pain, who suggested the pain medication, what it was, and how much they used.

They are then asked what they wanted the medication to do for them and what they wanted the medication to help them cope with or escape from.

Ask Patients

1. **What did you want the pain medication to do for you?**
2. **Did you get what you wanted?**

See the following table for the questions asked in this exercise.

Part 1: Your Personal Beliefs about Pain and Medication

1. Think back to the very first time you took any medication (including alcohol) for pain relief and write it like a story with a beginning, middle, and end. Make sure to include your age at the time, what you were doing, who you were with, what happened, what you were thinking about your pain, how you were affected (or feelings produced) by the pain, who suggested the pain medication, what it was, and how much you used.

2. What did you want the medication to do for you?

3. What did you want the medication to help you cope with or escape from?

4. What happened when you were growing up in your family when someone was in pain? What were the messages you received about pain management?

5. What's the most important thing you learned from completing this part of the exercise? What can you do differently for your pain management as a result?

Both Jean and Dean experienced several useful insights after completing this exercise. Jean was able to see how her father frequently pushed pills at her when she complained about even mild symptoms. As a consequence, Jean learned from a very young age that pain was to be medicated, not tolerated.

Dean learned that his pattern was that pain must be hidden and not expressed. He remembers being shamed and humiliated by his father when he cried after spraining his ankle at age five. This set up his pattern of self-medicating and then hiding that he was doing so from others. Both Dean and Jean were determined to learn how to stop their past self-defeating patterns.

Exercise Three, Part 2:
Pain Medication Problem Checklist

The next step in the assessment process is to determine the level of the addictive disorder (substance abuse or dependency). This is facilitated by Exercise Three, Part 2: "The Pain Medication Problem Checklist."

Denial is one of the major symptoms of an addictive disorder, but in the case of someone addicted to prescribed pain medication for a *legitimate* reason, the denial system can be difficult to intervene on. The Pain Medication Problem Checklist is designed to help work around this denial.

This instrument includes thirty "yes" or "no" questions using the addictive disorder criteria covered earlier, as well as the DSM-IV diagnostic criteria for substance abuse and substance dependency. However, they are rewritten in a way that is more patient friendly. You can review the following questions.

Pain Medication Problem Checklist

1. Do you sometimes take medication in a larger dose than is prescribed by your doctor?

2. Do you sometimes take the medication more frequently than prescribed by your doctor?

3. Do you ever mix other medication (including alcohol or over-the-counter medication) with your prescribed medication without your doctor's knowledge or approval?

4. When you're using pain medication (including alcohol) and other drugs, do you ever put yourself in situations that raise your risk of getting hurt, having problems, or hurting others? (This includes things like driving while using prescriptions, alcohol, or other drugs; taking care of small children; getting into arguments; skipping work; committing crimes; etc.)

5. Have you noticed that you need to take more medication than you used to in order to get the pain relief you desire?

6. When you use the same amount of medication all the time, do you experience a reduction in your pain relief, and are you tempted to increase the dose?

7. Have you ever felt sick or anxious (or experienced other withdrawal symptoms) when you suddenly stopped using your medication?

8. Have you ever used your medication or other drugs (including alcohol) to avoid withdrawal symptoms?

9. Have you ever hidden from (or not told) one doctor what you have been given by another doctor (or about use of over-the-counter medication)?

---

10. Have you ever had a persistent desire or made unsuccessful efforts to cut down or control your medication?

11. Have you ever used your medication (including alcohol) or other drugs to try to escape from or cope with a problem or situation that you didn't know any other way to deal with?

12. Has anyone else (a spouse, parent, brother, sister, boss, or friend) ever told you they thought you might have a problem with your prescription drug use?

13. Have you continued to use your medication despite having physical or psychological problems caused by the medication (for example impaired liver functions, loss of memory, irritability, or depression)?

14. Have you ever experienced legal problems due to substance-related issues (such as forging prescriptions or driving while taking your mood-altering medication)?

15. Have you ever used pain medication without really needing it for physical pain?

16. Have you ever used pain medication (including alcohol) to cope with uncomfortable feelings or to manage stress?

17. Have you ever thought that your prescription drug use was becoming problematic?

18. Have you ever seen a counselor or other professional for help with your prescription drug (or alcohol and/or other drug) use?

19. Have you ever let other people down whom you cared about because you were using pain medication (including alcohol) or other drugs and were in withdrawal?

20. Have your family members or friends ever been concerned about the type, amount, or frequency of the pain medication you take (including alcohol)?

21. Have you ever continued using pain medication (including alcohol) or drugs even though you knew they were causing problems or making existing problems worse?

22. Has a doctor or counselor ever told you that he or she thought you had a serious problem with pain medication (including alcohol) or other drugs?

23. Have you experienced depression or even thoughts of suicide while taking pain medication?

24. Have you ever attended any self-help meetings to deal with pain medication use or problems that occurred, at least in part, because you were taking the medication?

25. Do you ever use your medications to feel high (euphoria)?

26. If you were told you had to stop your pain medication because of a medical problem, would it be difficult for you to stop?

27. Have you ever lied to or mislead a doctor to receive more (or stronger) pain medication?

28. Do you feel deprived or even angry when you can't get your pain medication as quickly as you would like (or get enough of your pain medication)?

29. Do you ever find yourself making excuses to use more medication than was prescribed by your doctor?

30. Did you feel uncomfortable or have the urge to rationalize/minimize (or even lie) when answering any of the above questions?

Exercise Three, Part 3
Interpreting the Pain Medication Problem Checklist

The interpretation of the checklist follows in Part 3. It includes asking patients to score the number of yes answers in two segments and then to check their level or risk of addiction. See the exercise in the following table.

1. Count how many times you answered yes to any of the questions numbered 1 through 15. How many yes answers did you check? ———

2. Count how many times you answered yes to any of the questions numbered 16 through 30. How many yes answers did you check? _____

3. From your yes answers above, check the box below that most accurately describes your level or risk of addiction based on your answers to the Pain Medication Problem Checklist.

❏ **Low Risk for Addiction:** If you answered no to all of the above questions, you are probably at a low risk for addiction.

❏ **High Risk for Addiction:** If you answered yes to three or more of the questions numbered 1 through 15 and answered no to all the remaining questions, you may be at a high risk of becoming addicted.

☐ **Early-Stage Addiction:** If you answered yes to three or more of the questions numbered 1 through 15 and answered yes to between two and four of the questions numbered 16 through 30, you may be in the early stages of addiction.

☐ **Middle-Stage Addiction:** If you answered yes to three or more of the questions numbered 1 through 15 and answered yes to between four and seven of the questions numbered 16 through 30, you could be in the middle stages of addiction.

☐ **Late-Stage Addiction:** If you answered yes to three or more of the questions numbered 1 through 15 and answered yes to seven or more of the questions numbered 16 through 30, you are probably in the late stages of addiction.

4. If you believe that pain medication (including alcohol) and other drugs can do things for you that you can't do without them, you are probably psychologically and/or socially dependent on those substances.

5. If you believe that pain medication (including alcohol) and other drugs can help you cope with or escape from things you can't handle without them, you are probably psychologically or socially dependent on pain medication (including alcohol) or other drugs to cope with pain and to solve problems.

6. Do you believe that the results of the Pain Medication Problem Checklist accurately describe your current level or risk of addiction to pain medication (including alcohol and other drugs)?

☐ Yes ☐ No ☐ Unsure Please explain:

Jean and Dean both saw themselves as addicted before completing this exercise, and the results of their checklists validated their impressions.

Please note the discussion with patients that follows this exercise is much more important than the exercise itself. This exercise helps patients see clearly some of the problems they have as a direct result of chemical use. Even though Jean and Dean were not in denial about the seriousness of their addiction, they were both surprised about the extensive effect of their drug use.

Depression is another common disorder that impacts patients coping with chronic pain. In addition, the medication and/or withdrawal from the medication can lead to clinical symptoms of depression. This is another area where teamwork is essential. Referring the patient to someone who specializes in identifying and treating depression is important if that is beyond your scope of practice or experience. Consider reviewing Terence T. Gorski's new book, *Depression and Relapse: A Guide to Recovery*, for a more in-depth look at depression—especially depression with co-existing disorders.

Grief and loss issues must also be evaluated. A major part of the healing process for most chronic pain patients is identifying and grieving the loss of their healthy self and/or their prior level of functioning. In later chapters you will see how Jean and Dean addressed these issues.

Exercise Three, Part 4: Making a Decision to Do Something Different

In the final part of Exercise Three the patient is asked to list both the benefits and disadvantages of using pain medication by completing the following form. The final question asks the patient whether they think the benefits they expected from the medication were worth the pain and problems they experienced.

1. **Benefits**: List the main things that were better for you because you used pain medication (including alcohol and other drugs)?	2. **Disadvantages**: List the main things that were worse for you, or problems that you had because you used pain medication (including alcohol and other drugs).

- **Biopsychosocial History**

A complete assessment includes a biopsychosocial history and a trauma history. Whenever possible, previous healthcare providers, significant others, and/or family members should also be consulted when gathering this information. Family-of-origin issues and other traumatic situations can have a significant impact on treatment planning and treatment outcome.

In several instances, the literature reports that chronic pain conditions can restimulate posttraumatic stress disorders (PTSD). This was certainly the case for Jean and to a slightly lesser degree for Dean. As you will see in later chapters, this information makes a difference in treatment approaches.

Uncovering Axis-II Disorders

This part of the assessment can also surface symptoms of possible Axis-II personality disorders, as was the case for Jean and Dean. However, caution should be used here because the effects of medication and/or the withdrawal affects will often be similar to many of the Axis-II conditions. If these symptoms form an ongoing pattern that predates the medication use, has been present since adolescence, and continues after detoxification, then you are probably dealing with an Axis-II personality or developmental disorder.

Once the assessments are completed, clinicians can start to develop early treatment approaches. The most important factor to remember is that effective treatment planning depends on accurate in-depth evaluations that will produce successful treatment outcomes.

The next chapter will explore some early APM™ treatment interventions and discuss which approaches were used with Jean and Dean.

Assessments need to be ongoing throughout the APM™ treatment process.

It is also important to note that identification and assessments need to continue throughout the entire treatment process. It is crucial to revise or update the treatment plan as the patient progresses through the treatment program. The APM™ system is designed to facilitate the practice of ongoing assessments.

The following chapter describes the APM™ early treatment approaches. We'll start by looking at the detoxification process and its impact on pain management. You will also see how the APM™ system worked for Jean and Dean during their early treatment.

• **Call to Action for the Fifth Chapter**

It is time to summarize what you learned so far now that you have come to the end of the fifth chapter. Please answer the questions below.

1. What is the most important thing you have learned about your-self and your ability to help addicted pain patients as a result of completing Chapter Five?

2. What are you willing to commit to do differently as a result of what you have learned by completing this chapter?

3. What obstacles might get in the way of making these changes? What can you do to overcome these roadblocks?

Take time to pause and reflect, then go to the next page to review Chapter Six.

Early Treatment Approaches

• **Detoxification or Medication Taper Issues**

Neurotransmitters and Pain Suppression

Stimulation of certain areas of the brain can cause pain suppression. In the brain there are a variety of chemicals called neurotransmitters—substances that transmit information to the brain and body. Three neurotransmitters—enkephalins, serotonin, and endorphins—are known to be associated with pain suppression.

Analgesic treatments—treatments that prevent pain—are believed to be mediated by endorphins and enkephalins. Consistent with this understanding, it is now believed that opiates relieve pain because they are similar in structure to endorphins and enkephalins and therefore act upon the same sites in the brain and spinal cord as do these neurotransmitters.

The concern about using opiates repeatedly over a period of time is that they can ultimately reduce the brain's own natural pain-suppressant neurotransmitters, since they are so chemically similar in structure. The brain responds and adapts by slowing down production of its own *endogenous* opiates (the endorphins/enkephalins) with the repeated use of *exogenous* opiates. In a sense, the brain begins to adapt to the presence of an opiate drug by reducing its own natural source of pain-suppressing neurotransmitters. The result is that opiate medication can ultimately increase the sensation of pain via the brain's adaptive response.

> The Development of Hyperalgesia
> Due to Long-Term Opiate Use

Opiates are commonly used to treat moderate to severe pain and can be used over prolonged periods for chronic pain conditions such as those associated with cancer. In addition to analgesic actions, studies show that opiate administration can paradoxically induce *hyperalgesia.*

Hyperalgesia is an extreme sensitivity to pain that in one form can be opiate induced, but it can also be caused by damage to nociceptors (pain receptors) in the body's soft tissues. Hyperalgesia has also been demonstrated to be a cardinal sign of physical withdrawal from opioids in animal study models for more than thirty years, and recent empirical data exists to support its occurrence in humans.

Neurotransmitters and Withdrawal

When someone who abuses narcotic analgesics abruptly stops taking these drugs, they often experience a very hypersensitive, painful physical reaction. This is why the narcotic withdrawal syndrome can be so uncomfortable and painful. It takes time (approximately two weeks) for the brain to readapt from opiate medication that has essentially replaced its own pain-reducing capacity, back to its natural ability to make and use endorphins.

Because of the potential for physical dependency (meaning that the drug produces tolerance and a characteristic withdrawal syndrome upon abrupt cessation of use), opiate medications should only be used with the highest degree of caution in persons suffering from chronic pain disorders.

The question now is how and where to start treatment? This varies depending on the results of the identification and assessment process discussed earlier. However, effective treatment cannot be achieved if the patient remains on problematic pain medication (including alcohol). In the APM™ treatment system the first approach is usually detoxification or taper and stabilization.

Inpatient versus Outpatient

Sometimes at this stage of treatment, admittance to an inpatient program is required due to the quantity and/or types of medication being used. In other situations, an outpatient detoxification protocol or medication taper can be effectively implemented. Whatever method is used, it must be implemented with the team approach in mind where the patient is an integral part of the team. An empowered, involved patient is essential to obtain positive treatment outcomes.

In early treatment, a major difference between pain clinics and CD (chemical dependency) treatment centers involves medication and detoxification issues. Although many pain clinics withdraw their problematic patients from most psychoactive medication, some do not. Meanwhile, most CD treatment professionals believe that chemical dependency (addiction) is a chronic, life-threatening disease. Therefore, they conclude that the removal of all psychoactive chemicals is imperative for effective treatment. If the progression of the addictive disorder is not too advanced, an outpatient detoxification protocol could be used.

Even when there is agreement on detoxification as the starting point for recovery treatment, how that task is accomplished may vary. For most patients it can be dangerous to suddenly withdraw them from their medication without medical precautions. Often those precautions will include other medication to ensure a safe withdrawal. The use of different types of medication could be medically safe but to abruptly discontinue the medication is often extremely uncomfortable and painful for the patient.

Two Approaches for Detoxification

In addiction treatment centers there are basically two methods typically used for administering detoxification medication: (a) on an *as-needed* (or PRN) basis and (b) a *regular interval* administration. One drawback of the PRN method is that the patient remains in the self-medication pattern, while a drawback of option (b) is that it usually results in the person experiencing high levels of pain before each dose is due. Although physician prescription of analgesics in sufficient doses may be preferable, a compromise solution would consist of an as-needed order with a range of doses, depending on the person's level of pain.

In many pain clinics the *pain cocktail* method is used for withdrawing patients from the problem medication(s). This technique allows the gradual and systematic withdrawal of analgesics, opiates, or benzodiazepines.

The process involves combining the detoxification medication into a single mix that is given in a disguising mixture (such as cherry syrup). The mix is given only at fixed time intervals on an ongoing basis. The decrease in medication is achieved by gradually withdrawing the active ingredients, while keeping the total volume the same. The rationale for utilizing this method is that it is easier on the patient and the staff.

> Patients need to be proactive
> in their own healing process.

However, one difficulty with the pain cocktail approach is that it keeps the patient in a passive role. The APM™ approach encourages people to take a proactive part in their treatment, which includes being informed about the exact parameters of their detoxification protocol.

Detox for Jean and Dean

Now we will look at the approaches used when Jean and Dean went through their detoxification.

> Dean needed inpatient detoxification.
> Jean needed a medication taper protocol.

Dean's last relapse started with his abusing a nonsteroid, anti-inflammatory medication, Ultram®. This medication is contraindicated for patients with a history of opiate dependency/abuse, and in Dean's case it retriggered his addiction. In fact, it was shortly after starting the Ultram® (Tramadol) that he began to search out and use Vicodin again.

This retriggering effect for Dean resulted in visits to urgent-care clinics to receive Vicodin, which he started abusing in a short time and eventually buying it on the street again in large quantities. At the same time he was using a benzodiazepine (Xanax) medication for his anxiety. While in treatment after this relapse episode, Dean realized and admitted for the first time that he was using his medication for emotional pain as well as for his physical pain symptoms.

Dean's early treatment plan included not only detoxification and stabilization, but also training in emotional management skills. With Dean's combination and quantity of drug use, an addiction medicine practitioner determined that inpatient treatment was the safest modality.

> Jean's case was different.

Jean's motivation for treatment was also an external intervention. Her family insisted that she be in pain management treatment due to her significant problems that included being found unconscious by her young daughter due to overmedicating. Since she was not on that high a level of medication, Jean's healthcare providers were open to a medication taper while in the residential treatment program instead of completing a detoxification protocol first. One of her primary treatment goals was to eliminate opiate pain medication completely before leaving treatment.

This was very frightening for Jean, because she did not believe she could ever function without her pain medication—especially when experiencing a major pain flare-up. Since Jean's pain symptoms were amplified by a very toxic and stressful abuse history, one early approach included teaching Jean how to manage her stress and PTSD symptoms more effectively.

> Finding safer medication is crucial.

Ongoing use of pain medication can be a necessary treatment alternative for some patients. However, psychoactive medication such as opiates may be contraindicated for many chronic pain conditions due to the tendency for the user to develop tolerance. Earlier you learned about the importance of understanding the pharmacological implications for determining the proper medication for ongoing chronic pain conditions. Once again, it is important to emphasize that a team approach is crucial.

The importance of finding the safest medication protocol possible cannot be overemphasized. When the narcotic medication is taken in increasingly larger doses due to tolerance, the side effects from the medication may become physically and/or psychologically damaging and in some cases may become life threatening.

> Buprenorphine—A New Pain
> Management and Detox
> Treatment Alternative

There is now an effective medication for both opiate addiction treatment and/or maintenance pain management that was released since the original publication of this book. The new medication, buprenorphine, is an opiate agonist/antagonist and a very effective pain medication for appropriate patients. It has been used for pain management for many years, mostly in its injectable form. Buprenorphine is now available in the United States as sublingual (dissolved under the tongue) medication. It is many times more potent than injected morphine. Buprenorphine is different from other opiates, because the patient usually feels more "clear head-ed" when taking it.

It is the first oral medication that has been approved in the U.S.A. Physicians can now prescribe buprenorphine in their offices for people who are dependent or addicted to opiates, such as opiate pain medication, heroin, or methadone. Buprenorphine is an effective medication for opiate addiction that does not require daily or weekly visits to a clinic. Buprenorphine blocks the effects of other opiates; it eliminates cravings and prevents withdrawal symptoms such as pain and nausea. Patients can be maintained on buprenorphine or go through detoxification.

Subutex and Suboxone are new medications that have been approved for the treatment of opiate dependence. Both medications contain the active ingredient buprenorphine hydrochloride, which works to reduce the symptoms of opiate dependence. Subutex contains only buprenorphine hydrochloride. This formulation was developed as the initial product. The second medication, Suboxone, contains an additional ingredient called Naloxone to guard against misuse. Subutex is usually given during the first few days of treatment, while Suboxone is used during the maintenance phase of treatment. Both medications come in 2 mg and 8 mg strengths as sublingual tablets.

One significant drawback with this medication is that only qualified doctors with the necessary DEA (Drug Enforcement Agency) identification number are allowed to start in-office treatment and provide prescriptions for ongoing maintenance. Up until recently, prescribers were limited to a thirty-patient ceiling.

Fortunately, the Office of National Drug Control Policy Reauthorization Act of 2006 (ONDCPRA) modified the restriction on the number of patients a physician, authorized under the Drug Addiction Treatment Act of 2000 (DATA 2000), may treat—subject to the following conditions:

- Physicians must currently be authorized under DATA 2000.
- Physicians must have submitted the notification for initial authorization at least one year ago.
- Physicians must submit a second notification that conveys the need and intent to treat up to 100 patients and certifies their necessary qualifying criteria and their capacity to refer patients

for appropriate counseling and other appropriate ancillary services.

At the same time that the medication management issues are being decided, other treatment protocols must be developed. One major treatment intervention concerns stress and stress management.

• The Stress-Pain Connection

When patients are asked to give up their pain medication, an important early treatment strategy would be to teach them alternative methods of managing their pain. Patients should be taught simple stress reduction techniques that can be practiced during the detoxification period. It is important to educate patients about the connection between stress levels and their experience of pain and how stress management can decrease their suffering.

Learning to Identify Stress Levels

For Jean this segment of her work provided hope that eventual freedom from the medication was possible, but she also realized that it would be a difficult journey. Stress identification and reduction is an important tool for anyone recovering from chemical dependency and chronic pain.

When patients are aware of their stress levels, they can then take action to reduce their stress, which in turn leads to a decrease in their pain symptoms. Below is a reproduction of Exercise One, Part 4 from the *Addiction-Free Pain Management™ Workbook*, which both Jean and Dean utilized early in their treatment process to help them more accurately rate both their stress and pain levels.

General Stress Levels

Low Stress Level (stress score: 1–3)

    1 Very relaxed; vacation mode

    2 Stress is managed well; no discomfort

    3 No Notable distress or dysfunction

Moderate Stress Levels (stress score: 4–6)

    4 Higher stress levels: normal operating level, no distress

    5 Stress managed poorly at times; some discomfort but no distress

    6 Some notable distress but no dysfunction

Severe Stress Levels (stress score: 7–10)

    7 Very high stress levels

    8 Stress is usually managed poorly

    9 Stress causes notable distress and dysfunction

Score 7	=	I Space Out
Score 8	=	I Get Defensive
Score 9	=	I Overreact
Score 10	=	I Can't Function (or run away)

Learning to Measure Pain Levels

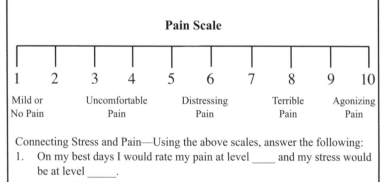

Think of a time when you were experiencing very low levels of pain and for some reason your stress levels went up. What happened to your level of pain? Most likely it also increased. Use the stress scale above and the pain scale below, using the 1-to 10-point rating system, when asked to describe your pain and stress levels.

Pain Scale

1	2	3	4	5	6	7	8	9	10
Mild or No Pain		Uncomfortable Pain		Distressing Pain			Terrible Pain		Agonizing Pain

Connecting Stress and Pain—Using the above scales, answer the following:

1.   On my best days I would rate my pain at level _____ and my stress would be at level _____.

2. On an average day I would rate my pain at level _____ and my stress would be at level _____.

3. On my worst days I would rate my pain at level _____ and my stress would be at level _____.

- **Support Systems**
Building Trust and Safety

Another potential block to effective treatment for Jean was her difficulty with trusting others and her resistance to using self-help groups. Finding the correct type of support system was not easy for her, but she finally chose a nearby women's group. Once she got to know the other women in the group, she reported feeling like she finally had a family-like group she might be able to trust.

Building trust and safety is a key part of any therapeutic process, but with the APM™ population it is even more important. Many times these patients learned that it was not safe to trust healthcare providers; many did not listen to their complaints or take their concerns seriously.

> Active listening leads to trust.

As discussed earlier, the APM™ approach encourages the use of active, compassionate, and empathic listening (strategically using same-word feedback) to facilitate trust-building with patients. However, it is important not to confuse compassion or empathy with sympathy.

Well meaning, sympathetic healthcare providers can sometimes come across as patronizing to patients with chronic pain conditions. These types of interactions support the perception of the APM™ patient as a victim of their condition. Jean was especially hypervigilant in this regard. Dean had his own issues with trust and safety, as well as isolation tendencies when his life became difficult.

Using Twelve-Step Support

While Dean was willing, and even eager, to use Twelve-Step support groups, Jean was very reluctant and believed she did not fit in at *those* meetings. Instead she chose a Christian recovering women's group. At first she was unable to open up and share. Later, when she felt safe and trusted the group, she actively participated.

On the other hand, Dean avoided his Twelve-Step support groups when he needed them the most. Their resistance was an important obstacle that needed to be overcome in order for Dean and Jean to be successful with their treatment.

Dean and Jean are not unique among addicted chronic pain patients who avoid Twelve-Step support groups. Many pain patients believe they are not *real addicts*, and therefore do not belong in Twelve-Step groups.

Well Intentioned but Dangerous Messages

Another obstacle facing pain patients, especially those who must remain on some type of medication, is that they often get confusing and conflicting messages at AA (Alcoholics Anonymous) or NA (Narcotic Anonymous) meetings.

The message they hear is that in order to "belong," you must stop using everything—no matter what. This is not the official position of either of these programs. However, advice from well-meaning recovering alcoholics and addicts can occasionally sabotage a pain patient's recovery process with all-or-nothing messages.

Precautions When Using Twelve-Step Support

There have been a number of patients with chronic pain and addictive disorders who have received inappropriate advice from their self-help recovery programs. These situations, which can be frustrating for patients and their treatment providers, have led others to relapse and, in some cases, death.

Patients referred to Twelve-Step groups must be informed that this may happen. They need to be prepared to deal with well-meaning people in recovery. It is helpful to refer patients to the Alcoholics Anonymous conference-approved pamphlet that clearly explains that some members need to be on *appropriate* medication.

Taking medication is a serious concern for someone in recovery, but as we explained earlier, sometimes medication is necessary for certain chronic pain conditions. This is where the Medication Management Components of APM™ are useful.

Using Pills Anonymous and
Chronic Pain Support Groups

There are other Twelve-Step programs that are often more appropriate for addicted chronic pain patients who develop problems due to pain medication use. One program is called Pills Anonymous (PA) and the other is called Chronic Pain Anonymous (CPA).

Other communities may have other chronic pain support groups that are also beneficial for APM™ patients. Group therapy and peer support have proven to be effective components for successful treatment outcomes and should be sought out.

Support groups and therapy groups also provide another essential component—nonpharmacological pain management suggestions and stress reduction tools. Both Jean and Dean were finally able to join and stay connected with appropriate peer support groups.

Another useful tool for someone in recovery from pain and chemical dependency is a twelve-item protocol developed by Dr. Stephen F. Grinstead and Sheila Thares, RN, MSN. The following tool was given to both Jean and Dean, who eventually used it very effectively. A full version of this tool is located in the Appendix of this book, but twelve of the recommendations are highlighted below.

A Guide for Managing Chronic Pain in Recovery
By Dr. Stephen F. Grinstead, LMFT, ACRPS
and Sheila Thares, RN, MSN

1. During early recovery postpone nonemergency dental work and elective surgical procedures that would require mind-altering medications. When you do need to be on medication, make sure that an addiction medicine practitioner/specialist is in charge of consulting about and/or prescribing that medication.

2. If you need to be on medication, have your sponsor, significant other, or an appropriate support person hold and dispense the medication. It would also be beneficial to only have a twenty-four-hour supply.

3. Consult with an addiction medicine practitioner/specialist about using nonaddictive medications such as anti-inflammatory, Tylenol, or other over-the-counter analgesics.

---

4. Be open to exploring all nonchemical pain management modalities. Some of the more common ones are acupuncture, chiropractic, physical therapy, massage therapy, and hydrotherapy. In addition, identifying and managing uncomfortable emotions may also decrease your pain significantly.

5. Be aware of your stress levels and have a stress management program in place such as meditation, exercise, relaxation, music, etc. If you lower your stress, you will usually lower your pain as a result.

6. Take personal responsibility to augment your support group meetings in order to decrease isolation, as well as urges and cravings.

7. Inform all of your healthcare providers about being in recovery, and be aware of the importance of consulting with an addiction medicine specialist in the event mind-altering medication is needed. There may be times you need to be on medication, but the risk of relapse can be minimized if open communication is maintained between the addiction medicine practitioner/specialist, yourself, and other healthcare providers.

8. Do not overwork, especially if you are in pain or sick. Take time off from work to heal and avoid fatigue.

9. Be open and aware of the cross-addiction concept. Any psychoactive chemical could trigger a relapse of your addiction.

10. As depression is common for people with chronic pain, be open to the possibility of taking appropriate antidepressants if needed.

11. Be aware of the importance of proper nutrition and exercise as an important part of chronic pain recovery. Stretch slowly at first, then structure progressive walking at least twice a day, increasing the distance as you are able. Add strengthening exercises if cleared by your healthcare provider. Remember, protein assists repair of injuries. Therefore, it is important to create a nutrition plan for tissue repair.

12. Explore your past beliefs and role models from childhood regarding pain and pain management. Look for healthy role models for pain management in recovery.

- **Exercise Four: Moving into the Solution**

Another useful tool to help patients avoid relapse early in treatment is Exercise Four in the *Addiction-Free Pain Management™ Workbook* titled "Moving into the Solution." This exercise includes a presenting problems report form, a relapse intervention plan, a medication management agreement, a craving management plan, and a nonpharmacological pain flare-up plan.

Part 1-A of this exercise asks the patients to identify current problems, list how the problem is connected to their inappropriate use of pain medication or self-defeating behaviors, and asks the patient for a commitment to stop. They are also asked to identify a situation in the near future that could cause them to start using pain medication inappropriately.

Part 1-B gives the patient a chart, shown below, to summarize the information. The intervention plan outlines the roles of the recovering person, the therapist, and at least three significant others. This exercise is reproduced below.

Both Jean and Dean had some difficulty in choosing appropriate significant others. It was also difficult for them to come up with effective intervention requests as they were so used to isolating and depending only on themselves. Fortunately, after several attempts, they were able to find supportive people who were willing and able to be an effective part of their relapse prevention network.

The other important parts of Exercise Four in the *Addiction-Free Pain Management™ Workbook* are shown in the tables that follow.

Exercise Four, Part 1-A: Presenting Problems

1. **Presenting problems:** What are the presenting problems that caused you to seek help at this time? (Why did you seek help now? Why not yesterday or next week? What would have happened if you didn't seek help now? What problems or negative consequences can this workbook help you avoid?)

2. **Relationship to inappropriate use of pain medication:** How is each presenting problem related to your inappropriate use of pain medication and/or to an ineffective pain management program?

    How is this problem related to your inappropriate use of pain medication (including alcohol) or other mood-altering substanc-

---

es? Did the chemicals cause you to have this problem? (i.e., Would you have this problem if you never inappropriately used pain medication, including alcohol or other drugs?) Did inappropriate use of pain medication (including alcohol) or other drugs make this problem worse than it would have been if you hadn't been using it?

3. **Consequences of not stopping:** What additional problems could you experience if you keep inappropriately using pain medication (including alcohol) or other drugs despite these problems? (What are the benefits? What are the disadvantages? What is the best thing that could happen? What is the worst? What is the most likely thing that will probably happen?)

4. **Asking for a commitment to stop (The Abstinence Commitment):** Are you willing to make a commitment not to inappropriately use pain medication (including alcohol) or other drugs for <name the specific period of time: _____>? (This should be done with the assistance of your doctor and counselor.) Please explain your answer.

5. **Immediate high-risk situations:** Are you facing any situations in the near future that could cause you to inappropriately use pain medication (including alcohol) or other drugs despite your commitment not to? Please explain your answer.

6. **The APM™ commitment:** Are you willing to make an agreement to complete the APM process to learn how to identify and manage those high-risk situations without inappropriately using pain medication (including alcohol) or other drugs?

   ❐ Yes ❐ No ❐ Unsure   Please explain:

Exercise Four, Part 1-B:
Presenting Problems Report Form

My Presenting Problems	Relationship to Inappropriate Pain Medication (Including Alcohol) or Other Mood-Altering Drug Use	Consequences If I Keep Using

Exercise Four, Part 2: The APM Medication Management Agreement

I, _____, do hereby agree to ABSTAIN from using any *inappropriate* medication (including alcohol) or other drugs and to continue an effective pain management program while I am completing this *APM Workbook*. Inappropriate medications are those that have not been authorized by my treatment team, and it includes prescription medications (including quantity and frequency of use), over-the-counter medications, as well as alcohol, and other mood-altering substances.

Should I return to using any inappropriate pain medication (including alcohol) or other drugs and/or deviating from my pain management program, I will immediately seek help from an appropriate treatment team member. I will also be open to having my treatment plan reevaluated and modified if determined necessary by my treatment team. This intervention may require transfer to a treatment facility for detoxification and/or stabilization before continuing with the *APM Workbook*.

I also agree to submit to random drug screens at the discretion of my treatment team. Unwillingness to submit to a breath, blood, or urine test will be interpreted as a clear indicator I have been using inappropriate mood-altering chemicals, including alcohol, and that I need immediate intervention.

I will consult with my treatment team regarding any medications prescribed to me by any physician, and I will not use **anything** that is not approved by my treatment team including over-the-counter medications.

Signature _____   Date _____

Signature of Witness _____   Date _____

Exercise Four, Part 3:
Your Relapse Insurance Policy

Relapse Intervention Plan: One of the goals of completing this workbook is to prepare you to quickly stop the inappropriate use of pain medication (including alcohol) and other drugs, or ineffective pain management, should it occur. This exercise is called Developing a Relapse Intervention Plan.

Factors that stop relapse quickly: Your response to relapse will be determined in large part by the following three factors: (1) what you were told will happen if you start inappropriately using pain medication (including alcohol) or other drugs or start mismanaging your pain management program; (2) what you can do to stop using pain medication (including alcohol) or other drugs and/or get back to using an effective pain management program is relapse occurs; and (3) the approach of the treatment professionals who deal with you after the relapse has occurred.

Guidelines that stop relapse quickly should it occur: It's a mistaken belief that if you take one dose of a drug, you will lose control and not be able to stop until you hit bottom. There are two reasons not to believe this: First, it's not true. Many chemically dependent people have short-term and low-consequence relapses and get back into recovery before serious damage occurs. Second, this approach programs you for a long-term catastrophic relapse episode. If you do start to inappropriately use pain medication (including alcohol) or other drugs, the misleading voice may pop into your head saying, "If you take one dose of a drug, you will lose control and not be able to stop until you hit bottom." You may then say to yourself, "Great, now I can keep medicating until I hit bottom." This does not mean it's perfectly fine to take single drug doses whenever the mood strikes or as long as your life doesn't fall apart. You still have to be vigilant. "Single dosing" is a high-risk situation. Fortunately, if you do start to inappropriately use pain medication (including alcohol) or other drugs, you will hit moments of sanity where you can choose to stop the relapse and get help. At these moments it is important to act immediately. If you wait, the urge to use again will come back and the opportunity will be lost. If you do start to use alcohol and drugs and hit a moment of sanity where you want to stop, the four most effective things for you to do are:

- Read your prepared relapse intervention plan, which should always be readily accessible. (You also should have given copies to significant others.)
- Immediately stop using and get out of the situation that supports inappropriate use of pain medication (including alcohol) and other drugs.
- Immediately call for help and get into a sobriety supportive situation.
- Call a counselor or sponsor, go to a treatment program, or get to a support-group meeting.

The Relapse Intervention Plan: In its simplest form, developing a relapse intervention plan consists of processing the following questions by developing a specific written plan in response to each question.

1. What is the counselor supposed to do if you relapse, stop coming to sessions, or fail to honor your treatment or abstinence contract?
2. What are you going to do to get back in recovery if you start inappropriately using pain medication (including alcohol) or other drugs so that you can stop using before you hit bottom?
3. Who are three significant others who have an investment in your recovery? What is each of them supposed to do if relaspe occurs? Make sure you have their day and night phone numbers accessible and they have a copy of this plan.

A. Name of Significant Other #1 _____
   Phone: _____

   What are they supposed to do? _____
B. Name of Significant Other #2 _____
   Phone: _____

   What are they supposed to do? _____
C. Name of Significant Other #3 _____
   Phone: _____

   What are they supposed to do? _____

Exercise Four, Part 4: Pain Management Craving Intervention Planning

Developing Your Personalized Craving Management Plan

When you have made a decision to take action and follow a healthy living plan and manage your pain in a recovery-prone manner, there is a strong possibility you may experience intense urges or cravings to once again use inappropriate medication (including alcohol and other drugs) to cope with stress or for pain relief and comfort. This doesn't mean you are weak or don't have a commitment to follow your Medication Management Agreement and recovery plan. It is normal for people who quit using medication inappropriately to have thoughts and even strong cravings to fall back into old ways.

You can avoid relapsing into old behaviors by creating an effective craving management plan. Below are ten examples of steps you can take to avoid giving into your cravings.

Directions: As you read each of the interventions below, rate **your** ability to implement each one on a scale of 1 to 10, with **1** meaning "I would probably not be able to do that" and **10** meaning "I could definitely do that."

Recognize and Accept: Recognize the craving and accept it as a normal part of your recovery. Remind yoursel: "Just because I'm having a craving, doesn't mean there is something wrong with me. It is normal to have cravings." _____

Decide Not to Act on the Craving: Tell yourself the following: "No matter what happens, I'm not going to act on this craving. Instead I'll call someone." And/or "Cravings go away whether I use or not. I have proven this before and I can do what it takes to shut this down." _____

Change Physical Setting: Change your physical and/or social location—**GET OUT OF THERE!** Sometimes something as simple as changing chairs makes a big difference. Don't be around negative people who pressure you to give into your cravings. Be around positive recovery-prone people. _____

Meditation and Relaxation: Learn simple relaxation and/or meditation techniques (your healthcare provider can help you with this). Sometimes just taking a few deep breaths can also make a big difference. Some people report great benefit from meditation and/or relaxation cassettes. Check it out! Remember, contempt prior to investigation equals ignorance. _____

Negative Consequences: Remind yourself of the negative things that will probably happen if you give into your craving and start to use again. Have this prepared before you start experiencing cravings. Remember all the pain and problems you have experienced and the pain your significant others had as a result of your giving into your cravings before. _____

Benefits of Not Using: Remind yourself of all the good things that can happen if you do not give into your cravings and adhere to your Medication Management Agreement. List some of the things that you can now accomplish because you are clean and sober that would have been difficult, if not impossible, to do while using. _____

Exercise: Have a regular daily pattern of exercise and other pain management protocols developed, and practice them consistently. When you have a craving, you can begin using one of these activities to help you better manage your cravings. _____

Eat Healthy: Eating three balanced meals per day with nutritious snacks in between will be very helpful. Avoid eating as a "substitution" for the using, but do fuel your body in a healthy way. Avoid sugar, caffeine, and nicotine as much as possible, especially when having cravings. _____

Mastery Imagery: Close your eyes and imagine yourself being successful and powerful by not giving into your cravings. Imagine all the positive benefits you will experience and how good you will feel about yourself for not giving into the cravings. _____

Do Anything Else that Works: You know yourself better than anyone else does, so use that knowledge to develop an action plan. You can be successful in handling urges and cravings. Allow yourself to succeed and improve the quality of your life. _____

My Personal Plan: Try to imagine yourself in a situation where you would begin to experience strong urges or cravings to use pain medication inappropriately, including alcohol and other drugs. Then using the above interventions as a starting point, list your step-by-step action plan in the space below. Your plan should be at least four (4) steps—but in this case more is definitely better.

When helping patients complete the craving management exercise, it is important to educate them about the connections between addictive thinking and uncomfortable emotions that lead to cravings. The following chart can help achieve that goal.

Feelings and Cravings

Feeling + Addictive Thinking = Craving

☐ Strong	or	☐ Weak	*Intensity* = ___
☐ Angry	or	☐ Caring	*Intensity* = ___
☐ Happy	or	☐ Sad	*Intensity* = ___
☐ Safe	or	☐ Threatened	*Intensity* = ___
☐ Fulfilled	or	☐ Frustrated	*Intensity* = ___
☐ Proud	or	☐ Ashamed	*Intensity* = ___
☐ Lonely	or	☐ Connected	*Intensity* = ___
☐ Peaceful	or	☐ Agitated	*Intensity* = ___

Exercise Four, Part 5:
Pain Flare-up Planning

Developing Your Personalized Pain Flare-up Plan

When you live with chronic pain, there will be times when your pain flares up. Sometimes you can determine why, and other times it comes as a complete surprise and you don't really know why. No matter why your pain flares up, you need to find safe, effective ways to cope with the amplified symptoms. This requires having a good plan in place. Those who fail to plan, plan to fail!

Below are several nonpharmacological (nonmedication) ways that other people have developed to manage their flare-ups. The important thing to remember is that you **can** intervene in a way that helps you regain effective pain management. Sometimes the intervention may need to be pain medication, but changing your medication protocols should only be done with your healthcare provider's knowledge and permission. This worksheet can support you to adhere to your Medication Management Agreement.

1. **Breathing and Relaxation:** When you are in a pain flare-up, your body's automatic reaction often includes a reflexive tensing response. This can lead to being unable to relax the focus of the pain, which results in increased muscle tension in these areas. It is important to consciously practice relaxing the affected

muscles. This will enable you to modulate your pain levels and bring the pain under control without increasing your medication. Using deep, slow breathing can help you soften and relax your overly tense muscles.

2. **Increasing Activity/Fitness:** When you experience pain flare-ups, you may become sedentary and avoid many types of activities. The two primary reasons for this are the pain itself and your own predictions (*anticipatory pain*) regarding the negative impact of the activity. Therefore, it is crucial to return to more nomal levels of activities, then slowly increase your stamina for physical activities to extinguish conditioned avoidance patterns.

3. **Diffusing/Reducing Emotional Overreactivity:** When you are experiencing intense uncomfortable emotions—especially about being in pain—your pain levels can actually intensify. Your emotions become like an amplifier circuit that increases the volume of your pain. It is necessary to practice specific methods of reducing this automatic process that occurs in the face of stressful triggers. As you do this, you will realize that you may not be able to eliminate those problematic emotional triggers. But you **can** learn different methods of reacting and managing your feelings.

4. **External Focusing/Distraction:** The more you focus on your pain, the more you actually intensify your experience of the pain. When you learn to shift and manipulate the focus of your attention in a positive way, your experience of the pain will be minimized. This can be accomplished by changing how you think and feel about your pain. You can then direct your attention to pleasant activities or tasks that take the focus off of your pain.

5. **Using Anything That Works:** When your pain flares up, there are many interventions that you can try. In addition to those listed above, you can use breathing, muscle relaxation, visual imagery, music, cold/heat, stretching, massage therapy, stress management, acupuncture, acupressure, TENS Unit, journaling, hydrotherapy, etc.

My Personal Plan

Try to imagine yourself in a situation where you are experiencing a pain flare-up and you want to intervene in a positive and proactive manner. Using the above interventions as a starting point, list your step-by-step action plan. Your plan should have at least four (4) interventions—the more the better.

This five-part exercise was a major turning point for both Jean and Dean. Both patients shared that the most important thing they learned was they could take action in order to manage their cravings. And, more importantly, they could develop a safe pain flareup plan. Jean shared her completed exercise with her church group and asked for their support in implementing it.

Dean shared his answers to these exercises with a close friend in his Twelve-Step program and gave key people permission to remind him of his commitment and plan. Dean believed it was also important to let his wife see his work, because that was a simple way he could start emotionally connecting with her. I reminded Dean that she was also one of his three relapse intervention team members, so she needed to know his plan in order to fully support him in a positive way.

Using Denial Management Counseling to Manage Resistance and Denial

When patients go through the exercises above, they are often motivated and encouraged in their ongoing recovery process. These exercises are part of the Denial Management Counseling approach that will be described in the next chapter.

Both Jean and Dean had made commitments to stop abusing their pain medications in the past, but this time they were encouraged to put it in writing. Both Jean and Dean shared later that having this signed contract helped them stop sabotaging themselves on several occasions.

Connecting Cause and Effect

For Jean it was important to finally connect that seeing herself as a poor parent was directly connected to her inappropriate use of pain medication. Once she realized what the problem was, she was more than willing to make a commitment to stop using her old coping behaviors.

Other early treatment approaches—the Nonpharmacological Treatment Processes, including nonpsychoactive pain medication, physical therapy, hydrotherapy, nonchemical pain management, and chemical dependency education—should be implemented when needed to facilitate detoxification and stabilization. These are some of the treatment approaches that are covered in the next chapter. It is important to remember that it is sometimes necessary to implement these interventions early on in the treatment process.

• Call to Action for the Sixth Chapter

It is time to summarize what you learned so far now that you have come to the end of the sixth chapter. Please answer the questions below.

1. What is the most important thing you have learned about yourself and your ability to help addicted pain patients as a result of completing Chapter Six?

2. What are you willing to commit to do differently as a result of what you have learned by completing this chapter?

3. What obstacles might get in the way of making these changes? What can you do to overcome these roadblocks?

**Take time to pause and reflect, then
go to the next page to review Chapter Seven.**

Chapter Seven
Utilizing Nonpharmacological Treatment Processes

Active versus Passive

Earlier we discussed the APM™ system being based on the concept that chronic pain patients require an active, multidimensional approach to obtain favorable treatment outcomes. Some chemical dependency treatment programs and many pain clinics have a tendency to put their patients in a passive role, which, as was demonstrated earlier, has proved to be counterproductive.

In addition to assigning a patient to a passive role, some chronic pain programs fall short as they lack a multidimensional approach. Corey and Solomon (1989) believe that chronic pain patients require an active, multidimensional approach to treatment. For example, the treatment plan might include exercises, chiropractic treatment, cognitive-behavioral strategies, and massage therapy. This combination is becoming known as multidisciplinary integrated pain management.

For many APM™ patients the first step needs to be helping them accept the need for recovery. This is where the CENAPS® Model of Denial Management Counseling (DMC) can be utilized.

• Denial Management Counseling

Denial Management Counseling (DMC) is a treatment modality designed to assist patients with alcohol and drug-related problems who have high levels of denial and treatment resistance. When the first edition of the professional guide came out, this process was still being called *Motivational Recovery Counseling.* But the new title, *Denial Management Counseling,* is more accurate as it uses a motivational recovery approach. Many APM™ patients need and benefit from this type of approach.

The DMC procedure focuses upon developing appropriate treatment plans, targeted interviewing, and using a sequence of proven action steps to gain an initial commitment to treatment.

Goals of DMC

- Interrupt the patients' denial
- Increase recognition of addiction-related life problems
- Identify the real problems and losses from drug use
- Motivate patients to accept referral to the next level of treatment

The *Addiction-Free Pain Management™ Workbook* incorporates a portion of the DMC process by using a medication management contract and decision-making exercises that were explained earlier. The new *Denial Management Counseling for Effective Pain Management Workbook* by Stephen F. Grinstead, Terence T. Gorski, and Jennifer C. Messier is an excellent resource for patients who need more comprehensive denial management work. Along with DMC, other treatment modalities need to be added at the same time to address the synergistic effects of the addictive disorder and the chronic pain disorder (i.e., the *Addiction Pain Syndrome*). In the following table is a list and brief description of the twelve pain-denial patterns from the *Denial Management Counseling* workbook, used with full permission.

Understanding and managing denial is crucial for effective pain management.

The Pain Denial Pattern Checklist

1. **Avoidance:** "I'll do anything not to talk about my pain management problems."
2. **Total Denial:** "No, not me! I don't have a problem with my pain!"
3. **Minimizing:** "My pain management problems aren't that big of a deal!"
4. **Rationalizing:** "If I can find good enough reasons for my problems with pain management, I won't have to deal with them."
5. **Blaming:** "If I can prove that my problems with pain management aren't my fault, I won't have to deal with them!"

6. **Comparing:** "Showing that others are worse off then me proves that I don't have serious problems with my pain management!"

7. **Compliance:** "I'll pretend to give you what you want so you'll leave me alone!"

8. **Manipulating:** "I'll play the game to convince others to do all the work for my pain management."

9. **Having a Flight into Health:** "Feeling better means that I'm cured and I can coast!"

10. **Fear of Change:** "If I don't focus on having a problem with my pain, I won't know who I am or how else to relate!"

11. **Diagnosing Myself as Beyond Help:** "Since nothing I do has ever worked for my pain management, I don't have to try anymore—I don't want to be let down yet again!"

12. **I Have the Right to Be This Way, AKA It's My Body:** "I have the right to whatever I want to do or don't do with my body and for my pain management, and no one has the right to tell me differently!"

- **Nonpharmacological Treatment Approaches**

Some of the following pain management interventions were briefly covered in Chapter Two. In the following pages you will have an opportunity to obtain a more in-depth overview of some of the most utilized nonpharmacological pain management interventions; there are many more approaches than can be covered here. In fact, the only limitation for incorporating new nonpharmacological interventions is your imagination and that of your patients.

Avoidance by Distraction

Throughout this book you have seen the word "denial" used many times. At this point it is important to interject that the psychological defense mechanism called denial can be problematic, but at times it may be helpful. Denial is problematic and can lead to life-damaging consequences when it is automatic and unconscious, leading people to avoid taking needed action. However, some denial patterns can be used strategically to help overcome problems.

One of these helpful patterns is a type of avoidance denial pattern called Avoidance by Distraction. This denial pattern can be used in a very positive way to help someone with their pain management. For example, I treated one client who learned to use this distraction tactic to focus on being present with her grandchildren instead of being overly caught up in her suffering. She discovered that when she was truly present with one of her grandchildren, she did not notice her pain as much. "Those who have something better to do, don't suffer as much" (W. Fordyce, Ph.D.).

Unfortunately, some people take the distraction to an extreme and end up causing more damage to their bodies as well as significantly increasing their pain levels. The goal here is to help people learn to focus their attention on something more interesting and positive than suffering. If you teach people to utilize this particular intervention, it would be useful to teach them proper activity pacing as well. Some people need to learn to slow down or take it easy, while others need to increase their activity levels and push themselves a little more.

Massage Therapy and Physical Therapy

One early pain management approach to consider is massage therapy. When using massage therapy, it is important to realize there will be some immediate pain relief and reduced muscle tension, but it will be short-lived if not followed with other measures. This is understandable since there are many precursors or triggers for muscle tension that often resurface soon after the massage session. Therefore, other measures must be implemented that are specific to the individual patient, and these must be used in the proper sequence.

Some of the methods that are successful in resolving these other precursors to pain are training the patients to use relaxation and meditation techniques, a customized exercise discipline, the use of biofeedback, and implementing proper nutrition, which is covered in a later chapter.

> Using Physical Therapy
> with Hydrotherapy

Many healthcare providers promote the combination of physical therapy and hydrotherapy to help patients learn how to strengthen and recondition their bodies, thus becoming active participants in their healing.

Reilly (1993) agrees that hydrotherapy and a water-based exercise program can be an extremely helpful, active modality for people with chronic pain. Because water buoys the body, the stress and strain is removed while in the water. Exercising in the water for short periods of time has benefits equal to several hours of land-based exercise, without some of the negative side effects.

Hydrotherapy and swimming were very important components of Dean's pain management program, especially because land-based exercise tended to be problematic for him.

TENS Units

TENS is an acronym for Transcutaneous Electrical Nerve Stimulation. With the development of modern medicine, doctors and scientists have perfected the use of electric pulses to treat and eliminate pain. TENS units use electro frequency at about 80 to 90 Megahertz. According to doctors and medical professionals, the TENS device is the most highly effective treatment for pain relief. Unlike prescription or over-the-counter drugs, TENS units are side-effect free when used as directed by a qualified healthcare professional.

A TENS unit transmits small square electrical pulses to the electrodes, which transmit this electrical pulse to the underlying nerves. The fundamental components of a TENS unit are the electrodes, a highly advanced computer chip, and an electrical battery source. A small amount of electricity is transmitted through the computer component then to the electrodes, which transmits the electrical waveform to the underlying nerves. The user can personalize the pulse frequency, which is the strength of the electrical current given to the electrode.

TENS units are prescribed for both acute pain and chronic pain conditions such as arthritis, joint pain, and fibromyalgia. For some chronic pain patients, a TENS unit provides pain relief that can last for several hours. For others, a TENS unit may help reduce the amount of pain medications needed. Some patients hook the unit onto a belt turning it on and off as needed. The cost of a TENS unit can range from about $100 to several hundred dollars. TENS units can be purchased or rented. A prescription usually is necessary for insurance reimbursement of a TENS unit.

Biofeedback

Biofeedback has proven to be another effective, active method that APM™ patients can learn, to further participate in their own treatment. Biofeedback is a treatment technique where patients are trained to improve their health by using signals from their own bodies. Physical therapists use biofeedback to help stroke victims regain movement in paralyzed muscles. Psychologists use biofeedback to help tense and anxious clients learn to relax. Specialists in many different fields use biofeedback to help their patients cope with chronic pain.

Devine (1988) discusses the condition of *dysponesis*, also called faulty bracing, where people tense up their muscles to pain thereby intensifying the pain experience. Dysponesis is defined by Doreland's Medical Dictionary as follows: "*A reversible physiopathologic state consisting of unnoticed, misdirected neurophysiologic reactions to various agents (environmental events, bodily sensations, emotions, and thoughts) and the repercussions of these reactions throughout the organism.*" One of the most direct methods for coping with dysponesis involves the use of biofeedback. This procedure teaches patients to let go of stress and tension.

According to Jaffe (1986) an effective biofeedback training program should be progressive and include several steps. The program starts with an accurate diagnosis of the problem followed by implementation of the proper treatment modality and time for the patient to practice in situations that simulate instances where the symptoms most often arise. Training the patient to use meditation and relaxation techniques to reduce stress would also be a helpful complement to the biofeedback process.

Hypnosis and Self-Hypnosis

Hypnosis has long been understood to produce varied effects in subjects. Although the public at large tends to associate hypnosis with stage performances and bad sitcom episodes, the medical community has approached the topic in a different vein. Originally viewed as a magical cure-all, hypnosis has undergone tremendous amounts of scientific testing in modern times. When used in an appropriate manner, hypnosis has proved to be an effective tool in the management of pain and pain perception.

Watkins and Watkins (1990) stated that the most common psychological explanation for how hypnosis works is based upon a dissociation model. This model has been seen in patients with a multiple personality disorder. Dissociation eliminates pain by placing it in a sort of psychological storage area, away from the primary consciousness of the patient. This model of dissociation is commonly referred to as the "hidden observer" model of cognition.

Wall and Jones (1991) believe that stress reduction practice, as well as other nonpharmacological approaches, combined with biofeedback, have proved to be an excellent way to reduce pain symptoms. Wall and Jones also discuss hypnosis and meditation as effective "belief and attitude" therapy approaches that have proved successful in treating chronic pain. Dean was open to hypnotherapy, especially learning self-hypnosis, to enhance his pain management.

> Self-hypnosis has proved
> effective for chronic pain management.

Self-hypnosis has also proved to be an effective tool for some patients' pain management programs. A major benefit is that it takes the patient out of a passive recipient role and makes them an active participant in their own healing. Self-hypnosis is a procedure where a patient is taught a simple technique to bring themselves to the alpha state, the place each of us goes every night just before we drift off to sleep. The difference, though, is that the patient does not sleep; instead, they experience a heightened state of awareness, where the "chatter" in the conscious mind is quieted and the subconscious mind is allowed to do what it does best—take care of the body. This opposite capacity of the body's reaction to stress has been called the alpha state, meditation, the sleep state, and the *relaxation response*. It is a conscious application of the body's innate ability to heal itself simply by relaxing.

The Emotional Link

Most chemical dependency treatment professionals realize the importance of teaching their patients how to deal appropriately with emotional issues to reduce their stress and anxiety. The Gorski-CENAPS® Model is based in part on the belief that avoiding painful emotions will often lead a recovering chemically dependent person to relapse.

Unfortunately, many pain clinics do not focus on the emotional component. In their review of thirty-two multimodal pain treatment programs, Corey, Linssen, and Spinhoven (1992) found many interventions and treatment approaches being used; however, none of those programs used emotional modalities. Fortunately, this is changing in some of the truly multidisciplinary, integrated pain management programs.

Corey and Solomon (1989) devote an entire chapter of their book discussing chronic pain and emotions. They explore the different treatment strategies needed to deal with emotions such as anger, depression, and anxiety. Some of the methods include cognitive-behavioral therapy exercises, as well as meditation and relaxation techniques.

Roy (1992) is another advocate of the link between chronic pain and emotions. Roy also believes in many cases, especially when there is clear and unambiguous evidence of suppressed or repressed emotional issues, that dynamic psychotherapy is an effective treatment modality.

Using the Twelve Steps to Manage Pain

Cleveland (1999) in her book, *Chronic Illness and the Twelve Steps: A Practical Approach to Spiritual Resilience*, maintains that dealing with the emotional component of chronic pain is an extremely effective treatment approach. Cleveland adapts and incorporates the Twelve Steps of Alcoholics Anonymous, showing people with chronic pain issues how to improve the quality of their lives and effectively deal with their emotions. Both Jean and Dean used Cleveland's book as part of their healing process.

Meditation

Dealing with emotions and promoting faster healing can be facilitated through the use of meditation. Meditation involves using any number of awareness techniques to quiet the mind and relax the body. Concentration practices and mindfulness meditation are perhaps the best known. Research shows meditation can help relieve many arthritis symptoms, such as physical pain, anxiety, stress, and depression, as well as ease the fatigue and insomnia associated with fibromyalgia. It affects many body processes connected with well-being and relaxation. Recent studies suggest meditation may balance the immune system to help the body resist disease and even heal.

> Meditation has proved effective
> in chronic pain treatment.

Khalsa and Stauth (2002) discuss in their book, *Meditation as Medicine,* the process of using an adapted version of Kundalini yoga and meditation to help the body heal itself. This process has also proved beneficial to assist patients in reducing their pain and suffering by committing to a daily structure of breathing and meditation.

Coffey-Lewis (1982) describes how the practice of meditation leads to true and lasting healing. Coffey-Lewis discusses how meditation takes on many different definitions for different individuals. For some, meditation is used for stress reduction; for others, it is a scientific way of interconnecting parts of the brain. Others find it helpful in healing the splits in personality and integrating wholeness.

Cleveland (1999) also promotes the use of meditation for improving quality of life and for self-healing. Meditation is also a part of the Twelve-Step process—the Eleventh Step. Reilly (1993) analyzes Step Eleven, showing people with chronic pain how to apply it towards their healing process, and demonstrates how to effectively use meditation. Both Jean and Dean spent a portion of many of their therapy sessions practicing breathing and meditation processes until they learned to automatically incorporate it into their daily schedules.

Evoking the Relaxation Response

There are many techniques and exercises for bringing about deep relaxation or the relaxation response. These include such things as breathing techniques, progressive muscle relaxation, visualizing a peaceful image, meditation, imagery, among others. In general, breathing exercises seem to be the easiest way to learn to elicit the relaxation response. They are probably the most appropriate initial technique to be used with chronic pain patients. The exercises are straightforward and require a minimal amount of body movement. This makes them easy to apply to most chronic pain conditions, even those in which restriction on movement or position may be part of the functional problem.

Caudill (2001) devotes two chapters in her book, *Managing Pain before It Manages You,* to the importance of evoking this relaxation response as an integral component of pain management. However, when explaining this to patients, it is important to distinguish the difference between the *relaxation response* versus simply *relaxing*. When discussing relaxation training as part of chronic pain management, patients often ask if they can simply do something they enjoy such as listening to music or sitting out in the backyard. It should be explained that although these types of activities are certainly relaxing, they do not elicit this relaxation response.

The type of relaxation that is important in chronic pain management is a form of deep relaxation. Deep relaxation, or the relaxation response, refers to a specific physiological state that is the exact opposite of the way the body reacts when it is under stress. The relaxation response was first described by Dr. Herbert Benson and his colleagues at Harvard Medical School in the early 1970s. It involves a number of physical changes, including a decrease in

- heart rate,
- respiration rate,
- blood pressure,
- skeletal muscle tension,
- metabolism rate and oxygen consumption,
- analytical thinking, and
- an increase in the alpha wave activity of the brain.

This type of deep relaxation or relaxation response can only be achieved with regular practice of a relaxation technique. Once the patient learns to elicit the relaxation response, they will notice feeling more relaxed even when not directly practicing the relaxation technique. The deep relaxation response also directly impacts the physical stressors associated with chronic pain. These include

- pain reduction;
- control of side effects to medications, such as nausea;

183

- enhanced immune responses that may keep the patient healthier; and
- improved respiratory function.

Dealing with Grief/Loss Issues

One of the most difficult, and most crucial, emotional issues that needs resolution for this population is their grief and loss of health and/or prior level of functioning. Many chronic pain patients have lost careers, relationships, homes, and friends; other quality of life areas have been severely impacted as well.

Psychotherapists who will facilitate the grieving process with their patients should be part of the APM™ team. A review of the works of Elizabeth Kubler-Ross on the grieving process is also helpful in this regard.

Grief work was an important part of healing for both Jean and Dean, but especially so for Dean. One of the reasons Dean used medication was to help him function at a higher level of physical activity. Unfortunately, when he was under the influence of the pain medication, Dean overextended himself and, in some cases, experienced new injuries that obviously increased the severity of his pain.

In addition, Dean had some serious shame issues regarding what determines a "real man," especially in the area of sexuality. In fact, this sexuality/shame issue was a major precursor to a previous divorce, as well as his tendency to have affairs. These issues were threatening his current marriage. For Dean, working through this grief/loss and shame was crucial to his avoiding future relapse episodes.

Acupuncture

Acupuncture is one of the oldest, most commonly used medical procedures in the world. Originating in China more than 2,000 years ago, acupuncture began to become better known in the United States in 1971 when *New York Times* reporter, James Reston, wrote about how doctors in China used needles to ease his pain after surgery.

The term acupuncture describes a family of procedures involving stimulation of anatomical points on the body by a variety of techniques. American practices of acupuncture incorporate medical traditions from China, Japan, Korea, and other countries. The acupuncture technique most studied scientifically, involves penetrating the skin with thin, solid, metallic needles that are manipulated by the hands or by electrical stimulation.

Corey and Solomon (1989) discuss both the positive aspects of acupuncture and the fact that some people experience no benefit or limited benefit from it. Another drawback of this procedure is that frequent acupuncture treatments encourage a patient's passive role in treatment, which is counterproductive to effective ongoing pain management.

Jean experienced no benefit from acupuncture and discontinued it after a few sessions. Dean experienced only limited relief at first, but acupuncture eventually became an important intervention to help him reduce his major pain flare-ups. Many chronic pain patients experience significant benefits from acupuncture. An NCCAM (National Center for Complementary and Alternative Medicine, 2004) funded study recently showed that acupuncture provides significant pain relief, improves function for people with osteoarthritis of the knee, and serves as an effective complement to standard care. Further research indicated that there are additional areas where acupuncture interventions are useful.

For example, promising results have emerged showing efficacy of acupuncture in adult postoperative and chemotherapy nausea and vomiting and in postoperative dental pain. There are other situations—such as addiction, stroke rehabilitation, headache, menstrual cramps, tennis elbow, fibromyalgia, myofascial pain, osteoarthritis, low-back pain, carpal tunnel syndrome, and asthma—where acupuncture may be useful as an adjunct treatment, included in a comprehensive management program, or used as an acceptable treatment alternative.

Cold Laser Therapy

The term "cold laser" refers to the use of low intensity or low levels of laser light. Proponents claim that cold laser therapy can reduce pain and inflammation. The U.S. Food and Drug Administration (FDA) considers these laser devices investigational (experimental) and allows them to be used in studies based on evidence that they provide temporary pain relief.

185

Cold laser treatment is thought to help some types of pain, inflammation, and wound healing. These lasers are used directly on or over the affected area. Well-controlled scientific studies are underway using reliable low-level laser devices for pain, wounds, injuries, and other conditions. Certain types of cold laser treatment may eventually become part of conventional medical care.

Cold lasers may also be used for acupuncture, using laser beams to stimulate the body's acupoints rather than needles (see Acupuncture, previously mentioned). This treatment regimen appeals to those who want acupuncture but who fear the pain of needles.

Chiropractic Treatment

Many chronic pain patients receive long-term pain reduction when undergoing chiropractic treatment. Chiropractic adjustments restore proper motion and function to damaged joints, thereby reducing irritation to associated muscles and nerves.

Most chiropractors are trained in nutrition and often include dietary changes and nutrient supplementation in their treatment plans. This process helps to build up the immune system while at the same time raising the patient's pain threshold. Later in this chapter you will learn about the importance of using supplements as part of the healing process.

> Chiropractic care works
> for many chronic pain conditions.

There are a number of published studies supporting the effectiveness of chiropractic care for several types of chronic pain. For example, a study by Milne (1989) reported that out of 150 patients suffering migraine headaches, 98 percent experienced immediate relief of migraine through adjustments of the neck and through traction. Since many people are prescribed potentially addictive medication for migraine relief, chiropractic treatment could be a much safer—and often a more effective—alternative.

The largest comparative study of its time on treatment of back pain (Meade, 1995) concluded that chiropractic care was the superior treatment for chronic low back pain. Some case studies on whiplash treatment (Osterbauer, 1992) suggest that chiropractic care is effective for relieving the chronic pain often experienced after these injuries.

Activator Methods®
Chiropractic Technique

One of the newer, scientifically based chiropractic procedures is the Activator Methods® Chiropractic Technique (AMCT). The AMCT is described by Fuhr (1995) as a process of analysis and instrumentation designed to monitor and affect the neuromusculoskeletal system. The implement that is used is the Activator Adjusting Instrument (AAI): a patented, hand-held adjusting device designed to generate reproducible and controlled results.

However, as Fuhr points out, this process requires chiropractors to become certified via examinations to ensure a level of proficiency needed for effective and safe outcomes. So far fewer than 10 percent of chiropractors have become certified.

Yoga for Pain Management

Living with chronic pain can be a cause of constant discomfort that attacks a patient's reserves of strength, energy, and feelings of well-being. Yoga is an ancient system developed in India that addresses the physical, mental, and spiritual aspects of the individual. There are many different forms of Yoga practice, each of which emphasizes different skills and goals. Using Yoga techniques for pain management can help minimize medication usage and help people lead a happier and fuller life.

Breathing • Relaxation • Meditation

Three of the best techniques for pain management are Yoga breathing, relaxation, and meditation. These three aspects of Yoga can distract the mind from pain, reduce the body's tension in reaction to pain, and provide an opportunity to *move through* the pain instead of resisting it.

The act of controlling the breath in Yoga reduces pain. The body has a natural phenomenon built in to the nervous system that keeps tension in the muscles on "stand by" when the lungs are full or pressurized. The muscles will relax upon exhalation, deflating the lungs. So lengthening the time of exhalation can help produce relaxation and reduce tension in the body.

Yoga works on the body to reduce or eliminate pain by helping the brain's pain center regulate the controlling mechanism located in the spinal cord. Yoga also assists the brain with secretion of natural painkillers through the body. The potential benefits of Yoga in pain management have begun to be documented. Studies have shown its positive effect on stress through a decrease in serum cortisol levels and an increase in brain alpha and theta waves. It may also be of benefit by increasing self-awareness, relaxation on physical and emotional levels, respiration, and self-understanding.

Movement Therapies for Improved Pain Management

Tai Chi and Qigong

Tai Chi and Qigong are gentle movement practices that have been used for centuries in China for health, religious practice, and self-defense. As a form of exercise and relaxation, they have been used to improve balance and stability, reduce pain and stress, improve cardiovascular health, and promote mental and emotional calm and balance. Attitudes toward the basis of Tai Chi and Qigong vary markedly. Most Western medical practitioners, many practitioners of traditional Chinese medicine, as well as the Chinese government view Tai Chi and Qigong as a set of breathing and movement exercises with benefits to health through stress reduction and exercise. Others see Tai Chi and Qigong in more metaphysical terms, claiming that breathing and movement exercises can influence the fundamental forces of the universe.

In the area of pain management, scientific studies have shown their benefit in reducing stress, as evidenced by alpha and theta brain wave increases, increases in B endorphin levels, and decreases in ACTH (Adrenocorticotropic hormone) levels. Effectiveness has also been shown for complex regional pain syndrome, fibromyalgia, and chronic low back pain when combined with education and relaxation training. Studies continue to clarify the mechanisms of action, benefits, and applications of these movement practices for health maintenance and disease management.

- **Developmental Model of Recovery Transition and Stabilization Tasks**

Once patients are engaged in treatment and being withdrawn from the problem medication, they are in what the Gorski-

CENAPS® Developmental Model of Recovery refers to as the Transitional and Stabilization Stages of Recovery that we covered earlier.

According to this model there are four important tasks that need to be accomplished during these stages:

- Recovering physically from the withdrawal effects of chemicals
- Discontinuing a preoccupation with chemicals
- Learning to solve problems without using chemicals
- Developing hope and motivation for recovery

Stephanie Brown's (1989) Transitional Stage in like manner includes four tasks:

- Surrendering (hitting bottom)
- Forming of a new identity as an alcoholic and/or addict
- Discovering healthy behaviors to replace the addiction
- Learning relapse prevention strategies and abstinence skills

To give the APM™ patients the best hope of rapidly accomplishing these transitional tasks, they need to be quickly integrated into a treatment milieu. It is at this point that the DMC process, which was covered earlier, can be effectively implemented.

> APM™ patients fit in
> by attaining trust and safety.

Building trust and safety is crucial in order to help these patients fit in and bond. Many patients have learned to distrust others as a result of their dysfunctional family systems. By the time they enter treatment many patients have become isolated or may be exhibiting paranoid and/or agoraphobic symptoms.

Assisting the APM™ patients to work through their denial and other defenses using the DMC process, while at the same time supporting them to trust others, enables the pain patient to admit and begin to accept their substance use disorder. They can then identify with others in the treatment program or support groups and transition into a stable recovery.

Much of this process can be accomplished using group therapy followed by individual sessions on an as-needed basis.

From Victim to Empowerment

Since one component of this population's preoccupation with medication usually stems from an appropriate need for pain reduction, nonpharmacological pain treatment modalities are developed and put into place. An important goal during this phase of treatment is to begin empowering patients by supporting them to transition out of a passive role in dealing with their pain. It is crucial to assure them that a proactive approach, including the above modalities and other cognitive-behavioral strategies, can be successfully implemented.

There are many other alternative nontraditional pain management modalities that a trained treatment team can prescribe and implement as indicated by each patient's specific needs. Some of these *nonpharmacological treatment processes* were covered in the earlier part of this chaper. All the chosen strategies can then become an integral part of the patient's relapse prevention plan, which is covered later.

> APM™ uses an individualized
> nonpharmacological team approach.

An important point to consider is that the traditional "cookie-cutter" approach never did deliver positive treatment outcomes with the *usual* chemical dependency patient. Therefore, with the significantly more complicated problems that occur with chronic pain conditions (the Addiction Pain Syndrome), the approaches used must be individualized as well as wide-ranging. To that end, teamwork among all healthcare providers is essential.

> Nutrition and Exercise

• Nutrition and Healing

Up until recently there was a lack of information and a great deal of misinformation regarding the role of proper nutrition for effective pain management. The purpose of this section is to introduce you to some of the methods used as a part of the APM™ treatment approach. Recent research studies by the National Fibromyalgia Association (NFA) have confirmed that diet and nutrition play a significant and important role in the management of pain. The NFA

(2006) reports that success relies on utilizing a multidisciplinary and multidimensional approach, incorporating lifestyle and dietary changes to achieve optimum health and well-being.

The NFA also states that nutritional therapy practitioners are successfully using diet to treat and prevent illness and restore the body to a natural healthy equilibrium. Some healthcare practitioners believe that deficiencies of minerals and vitamins could be responsible for much disease and weakness in the body. Examples of conditions resulting from deficiencies include fatigue, lethargy, and susceptibility to colds and viruses.

The important role of proper diet and exercise as a part of addictive disorder recovery has been recognized for a long time. There is a significant amount of information about this in the recovery literature, such as the books *Passages through Recovery* (Gorski, 1989) and *Staying Sober* (Gorski and Miller, 1986).

There is also substantial pain management literature emphasizing the importance of nutrition and exercise in the healing process and effective pain management. In fact, Dr. Margaret Caudill (2001) devotes an entire chapter of her book, *Managing Pain Before It Manages You*, to the importance of nutrition in an effective pain management program.

> Nutrition impacts healing.

Later on, we will discuss and suggest some effective diet and exercise treatment plans and review the plans developed by Jean and Dean. Since in-depth coverage of nutrition and exercise is beyond the scope of this book, you will be introduced to several resources for additional research and information in the Appendix. You may also consider obtaining referrals to appropriate nutritionists in your area. Be sure to have consent releases signed to facilitate teamwork, treatment planning, and effective follow-up.

Nutrition and Pain
Foods That Help or Hinder

Murray and Pizzorno (1991) state that diet has little effect on a person's experience of pain, but it probably influences pain perception by the way it is associated with inflammation.

When metabolized, some fats and fatty acids may have a tendency to intensify the inflammation response, so their intake should be closely monitored. In addition, some foods act as triggers for certain pain conditions, such as migraine headaches.

Some of the problem substances that are linked to increases in pain are caffeine, alcohol, monosodium glutamate (MSG), and aspartame (NutraSweet®). On the other hand, some foods have been credited with pain reduction. Caudill (2001) reports foods linked to a decrease in pain include vegetarian diets as well as diets high in complex carbohydrates and low in protein.

Using a Food Diary

The use of a food diary can be beneficial in discovering which foods are part of the problem or part of the solution. For optimal success this should be done under the supervision of a doctor or nutritionist.

Ford (1994) reports that consumption of bioflavonoids, as found in fresh cherries, as well as eating other foods such as vegetables, legumes, whole grains, and some types of nuts can supplement some of the vitamins that seem to be deficient in people with chronic pain. However, caution must be used when taking vitamin and mineral supplements, especially with the tendency of chronic pain patients to use megadoses—the mistaken belief being that if a little is good a lot is better. Two conditions that seem to respond well to dietary changes are rheumatoid arthritis and gout.

The Naturopathy Controversy

Proper nutrition plays an important role in the art of *Naturopathy* (nature cure). Naturopathy is not universally accepted by the traditional medical society but has proven effective for many people.

Traditional naturopaths do not diagnose or treat disease, but instead focus on health and education. They teach clients how to create an internal and an external environment that is conducive to good health, enabling the clients to make their own choices. Naturopathy is based on the belief that the body is self-healing. The body will repair itself and recover from illness spontaneously if it is in a healthy environment. Naturopaths have many remedies and recommendations for creating a healthy environment so the body can spontaneously heal itself. The philosophy of naturopathic healing is based in part on the following:

- Discover and eliminate the primary cause of pain.
- Use the most natural, nontoxic, and least invasive therapy possible.
- Treat the whole person.
- Teach the person to develop a healthy diet.
- Support the body's own healing abilities.

Recent studies provide significant information and scientific data to ensure the safety and effectiveness of some naturopathic remedies. Although as Murray and Pizzorno (1991) point out, some therapies using colonic irrigation may be dangerous and lead to unwanted side effects, such as infections. Dr. Stephen Barrett (2006) suggests that a closer look at naturopathy's philosophy will show that it is simplistic and some of its practices are riddled with quackery.

Importance of Weight Management

Another important reason for good nutrition is weight management. Many chronic pain conditions become worse the more weight a patient gains.

Catalano and Hardin (1996) discuss how gaining weight can lead to a rise in back pain and increase the pressure on degenerative joints; whereas, being underweight can lead to an impaired immune system and frequent illnesses. This is one of the reasons APM™ incorporates nutrition and exercise into every treatment plan.

The human body functions most effectively at its optimal weight.

While Dean was near his optimal weight, Jean needed some additional interventions to help her reduce her weight by about forty pounds. The extra weight made it difficult for Jean to want to exercise, due to her fear of being judged by those watching her. In addition to a proper food plan, a prescription to join a hydrotherapy class that catered to overweight patients was the turning point for Jean. As she began to lose weight, her pain started to decrease, and her self-esteem and motivation to take care of herself increased.

Herbal and Homeopathic Remedies

Some chronic pain practitioners use the pain-relieving effects of herbs as an adjunct to a healthy nutritional plan. Murray (1995) states that according to the World Health Organization, about 80 percent of the world uses herbal remedies.

For example, the science of herbs is at the core of Chinese medicine. Also, a significant percentage of pharmaceutical products in the United States contain ingredients from plants. Fortunately, there has been an increase in research on herbal remedies, several of which have proven beneficial with negligible side effects.

On the other hand, some herbs have been found to have serious—and in some cases lethal—side effects. The vast majority of homeopathic medicines are also derived from plants, but before a remedy can be recognized as an official homeopathic medicine, it must be tested scientifically on healthy humans under a double-blind procedure to determine safety and effectiveness.

> ## Homeopathy—
> ## Science or Pseudoscience?

Homeopathy holds to the premise of treating the sick with extremely diluted agents that, in undiluted doses, produce similar symptoms in healthy individuals. Its adherents and practitioners assert that the therapeutic potency of a remedy can be increased by serial dilution of the drug, combined with what homeopaths call *succussion*, or vigorous shaking of the remedy.

Not altogether unlike conventional medicine, homeopathy regards diseases as *morbid derangements of the organism*. Homeopathy views a sick person as having a dynamic disturbance in a hypothetical *vital force*, a disturbance that homeopaths claim underlies standard medical diagnoses of named diseases. However, it is important to note that critics describe homeopathy as a pseudoscience and quackery. They claim the theory that extreme dilution makes drugs more powerful is inconsistent with the laws of chemistry and physics.

• Exercise and Healing

Most people will readily agree that regular exercise is good for you, and when combined with a healthy diet it will help people gain or lose weight, and generally improve their quality of life. Unfortunately, many people with a chronic pain condition mistakenly believe that they can no longer get the full benefits of exercise. Egoscue (1998) is very adamant that flexibility and mobility are the keys to successful pain management.

Type, Frequency, and Style

Exercise can and should be part of all pain management plans. The type and frequency of exercise is the important factor that requires someone with experience and clinical skills to develop an effective—and safe—program. Rest and immobilization periods (or uptime and downtime) should also be an integral foundation of the plan.

Other important considerations include the style of exercise, the progression of intensity, the frequency or quantity, and the prevention of additional injury. As mentioned earlier, hydrotherapy and water exercises can be very beneficial for people with chronic pain issues.

Most treatment providers working with pain management believe that mobilization through exercise is an important component of a successful treatment plan. Exercise helps increase range of motion, which is essential for increasing mobility and healing.

As mentioned earlier, the development of an exercise program should be done under the direction of a specialist. For some this will be their doctor, chiropractor, physical therapist, and/or personal trainer. Whichever specialist is chosen should become a part of the APM™ treatment team. Effective communication should be ongoing due to the exercise challenges that may occur with an APM™ patient.

Using an exercise specialist is important.

Using an appropriate and trained exercise specialist is important due to the different types of pain issues involved, as well as the different types of exercise modalities available to choose from.

Three Types of Exercise
Isotonic—Isometric—Isokinetic

There are basically three types of exercise, and each type achieves different results. The first type—isotonic—is active muscle contraction, moving a joint partially or thoroughly through its range of motion. Some examples of isotonic include flexing and extending various limbs, with or without using resistance.

The second type is also an active exercise—isometric—where the joint remains still during the muscle contraction.

The third type—isokinetic—is where resistance is applied to force muscles to exert maximum force throughout the range of motion. Isokinetic exercise requires specialized equipment.

Caudill (2001) discusses the importance of aerobic exercise at least three times a week to improve health and weight management. Many people with pain are afraid that their pain will increase if they become too active. However, the risks of not exercising far outweigh the fear of what "might" happen as a result of developing an exercise regime. Caudill states that if people are careful and progress slowly, they are not likely to worsen their condition.

Some of the forms of exercise recommended by Dr. Caudill include the following:

- Water exercise
- Stationary bike
- Treadmill
- Walking
- Yoga or Tai Chi
- Indoor cross-country ski equipment

When removing the pain is not possible, using exercise can increase a person's level of functioning, and thus improve their quality of life, enabling them to more effectively manage the pain. As mentioned earlier, Egoscue (1998) believes that flexibility and mobility are the best pathways towards reducing debilitating chronic pain. Another benefit of exercise is the increased ability of the body to produce additional endorphins. As we discussed earlier, these neurotransmitters help the body manage pain.

Catalano and Hardin (1996) note the fact that people who gradually incorporate exercise into their pain-management treatment plan return to a higher level of functioning and maintain more effective pain management. They also recommend a program of exercise that includes proper posture and stretching. Catalano and

Hardin show a secondary gain for exercise—reducing isolation tendencies.

Using Exercise to Socialize

As mentioned in an earlier chapter, isolation tendencies are common for people with chronic pain. Such was the case for both Jean and Dean. Jean used her hydrotherapy and water exercise classes as a place to socialize and share with people in a similar situation. Dean tended to socialize much less than Jean, but he was able to form a few close relationships with people who frequented the health club he joined.

Exercise and Stress Reduction

Reducing and managing stress is an additional reason for exercise. As discussed earlier, both Jean and Dean noticed a high correlation between stress and the intensity of their pain symptoms. Each of these patients used their exercise program as an integral part of their stress management strategy.

Dean noticed that if his stress levels were above a level seven and he could go swim a few laps, he could bring his stress level down to a four or five and was then able to manage it effectively. He also noticed that the distress he experienced as a result of his pain symptoms decreased at the same time.

In addition to effective stress management, Jean used exercise to help reduce her weight and increase her energy level. She noticed that after she gained weight, her pain symptoms increased. When she began a proper diet and exercise program, she reduced her weight and her pain symptoms decreased.

Exercise and Depression

As mentioned earlier, depression is common for people who live with a chronic pain condition. Managing depression is another important reason for a person with chronic pain to exercise.

Many therapists who work with various depressive mood disorders note that a regular exercise program is an important component of the treatment plan, but point out that additional measures may be needed. These measures could include nutritional changes and even antidepressants in some appropriate cases.

Diet and Exercise for Healthy Recovery

In addition to being an important part of an effective pain management program, a proper nutrition and exercise plan are essential components of a chemical dependency recovery plan. When people use psychoactive chemicals for a prolonged period of time, biochemical changes occur. Some of those changes were discussed earlier.

When people stop using drugs—whether it be prescription medication, alcohol, or other drugs—they often experience withdrawal symptoms. Fortunately, those symptoms are fairly short lived, from between three days to five or six weeks. Unfortunately, what follows is a period of protracted or post acute withdrawal (PAW). PAW can last between eighteen months to three years. The symptoms of PAW will be discussed in the next chapter.

Effective management for PAW includes a healthy nutritious diet and regular exercise. Also, the risk of relapse decreases significantly when people have an effective pain management and recovery program in place.

A proper nutritional and exercise plan needs to be a part of the APM™ patient's recovery plan, which is also covered in the following chapter.

> Nutrition and exercise are essential
> components of relapse prevention.

An ongoing practice of healthy nutrition and exercise can be a challenge to accomplish, but not impossible. Over a long period of time a patient's motivation may diminish, being replaced with boredom, forgetfulness, and distractions. However, having an effective relapse prevention plan in place that includes the nutrition/exercise dyad, along with the other components covered in the following chapter, will significantly decrease tendencies towards self-sabotage.

As discussed earlier, the *Addiction Pain Syndrome* produces a synergistic effect, so it is especially important to use a multidimensional treatment plan. This chapter emphasized the importance of combining the Nonpharmacological *Treatment Processes* with *Medication Management Components*. The next chapter covers the importance of using a relapse prevention plan that treats the synergistic effects of the Addiction Pain Syndrome. This process is called Reciprocal Relapse Prevention. You will also learn how Jean and Dean completed APM™ Core Clinical Exercises Five and Six.

- **Call to Action for the Seventh Chapter**

It is time to summarize what you have learned now that you have come to the end of the seventh chapter. Please answer the questions below.

1. What is the most important thing you learned about yourself and your ability to help addicted pain patients as a result of completing Chapter Seven?

2. What are you willing to commit to do differently as a result of what you learned by completing this chapter?

3. What obstacles might get in the way of making these changes? What can you do to overcome these roadblocks?

**Take time to pause and reflect, then
go to the next page to review Chapter Eight.**

Reciprocal Relapse Prevention

- **The CENAPS® Model of Relapse Prevention**

Because chronic pain is such a serious problem for many recovering people, often leading them to relapse, this stage of treatment is crucial for this population.

Over the past decade relapse prevention planning has become an important component in a number of chemical dependency treatment programs. Many programs now use the CENAPS® Model of relapse prevention developed by Terence T. Gorski—an innovative and dynamic process.

This method includes identifying high-risk situations for relapse, training in analysis and management of high-risk situations, developing a relapse prevention network, and constructing an early intervention plan to be implemented if serious signs of relapse appear.

Unfortunately, a literature review did not reveal any medical model pain clinics incorporating intensive relapse prevention plans into their treatment programs. However, some innovative pain programs that use a biopsychosocial approach do include some relapse prevention.

> Relapse prevention planning is a critical component of the APM™ treatment plan!

This chapter will illustrate and explain the relapse prevention protocols used with Jean and Dean. This chapter also reviews the exercises from the *Addiction-Free Pain Management™ Workbook* and shows how Jean and Dean completed that portion of their relapse prevention and recovery planning work.

- **Redefining Relapse**

Progressive Nature of Relapse
From Stability to Dysfunction

Relapse education must start with a new definition of relapse:

> Relapse is a progressive series of events
> that takes an individual from stable recovery to a
> state of becoming dysfunctional in their recovery.

The relapse process is marked by predictable and identifiable warning signs that begin long before alcohol and drug use or collapse occurs. This makes intervention possible for some clients before inappropriate medication use begins (including alcohol or other drugs). The appropriate response to relapse is to stop the relapse quickly by using a preplanned intervention, stabilize the patient in the appropriate level of care, assess the factors that contributed to the relapse, revise the recovery plan, and get the person back to working a personal recovery plan as quickly as possible.

When someone starts on the slide to relapse, they undergo many changes. The first change occurs in their thinking. Recovery-prone positive thinking is replaced by relapse-prone negative thinking and euphoric recall. Euphoric recall is remembering how good taking the pain medication used to be and self-talk about how awful it is not to be able to use now.

This negative thinking leads to a person experiencing uncomfortable and/or painful emotions. These feelings produce self-defeating urges, which are often followed by self-destructive behaviors. Inappropriate use of pain medication may not be an option in the early stages of relapse, but the negative behaviors often lead a person to experience more problems.

Relapse and Post Acute Withdrawal

One of the biggest relapse triggers for someone in early recovery is their inability to recognize and/or cope with the serious symptoms of protracted or post acute withdrawal (PAW). PAW is a series of biological and psychological symptoms that everyone in chemical recovery goes through. The brain chemistry is adapting and healing from the long-term toxic effects of alcohol/drug use. Remember in Chapter One this toxic effect was called *Substance-Induced Organic Mental Disorders*.

> ## There are six major symptoms of PAW:
> - Cognitive changes
> - Emotional changes
> - Sleep disturbances
> - Short-term and long-term memory problems
> - Physical coordination problems
> - An increased sensitivity to stress

When someone is also experiencing chronic pain, post acute withdrawal symptoms are often amplified by the accompanying stress of that condition.

• Relapse Prevention Planning

Relapse prevention starts with assessment and treatment planning followed by a high-risk situation identification process. High-risk situations for people with chronic pain are events that create an urge to use inappropriate pain medication or other drugs (including alcohol) after making a commitment to work an effective pain management program and use only approved medication exactly as prescribed. They also include situations that make patients want to stop using an effective pain management program despite their promises to themselves to lead a healthy lifestyle.

Identifying and Managing Core Issues

Besides core psychological issues and core addiction issues, APM™ patients also contend with core pain issues. Core pain issues are problems caused by the chronic pain condition and the patient's response to that condition. An example of a core pain issue is the cyclical increase (flare-up) of pain due to the stresses of everyday living.

Core addictive issues are problems caused by the addiction itself that would not exist if the addiction had not developed. They create emotional pain and dysfunction in recovery and require a recovery plan. Denial is a prime example of a core addictive issue, and, in the case of chronic pain patients, denial is often much stronger. A typical APM™ patient might say, "I can't be a real addict because I have a real pain condition and a doctor gave me the meds." Both

Jean and Dean identified this type of denial as one of their mistaken beliefs.

Core psychological issues are repeating problems caused by unresolved issues from childhood or unresolved adult trauma. They create a deeply entrenched system of irrational beliefs and coexist with the core addictive issues. Some common examples are post-traumatic stress disorder (PTSD), depression, and Axis-II personality disorders. In fact, a chronic pain condition will often retrigger PTSD. This is an area where a trained psychotherapist can have the greatest effectiveness.

Relapse Justifications

Relapse justifications are patterns of irrational thinking that create an immediate justification for chemical use. There are four common/basic justifications:

- **Euphoric recall:** ("It worked in the past so it must be OK now.")
- **Awfulizing sobriety:** ("Sobriety is and always will be a terrible struggle.")
- **Magical thinking:** ("This time I know using chemicals will fix me.")
- **Low tolerance for frustration:** ("I can't stand feeling so bad about….")

One of the most common relapse justifications for chronic pain patients is: "I have a legitimate reason to be in pain; therefore, it's OK to do anything I can to stop my pain." It is critical to teach patients how to identify and talk back to their relapse justifications and how to manage their warning signs or high-risk situations.

Exercise Seven (Analyzing and Managing High-Risk Situations) in the *Addiction-Free Pain Management™ Workbook* is an ideal tool for teaching patients to challenge old ways of coping as well as developing recovery-prone action plans. This exercise will be described later in the chapter.

The Relapse Prevention Network

For effective warning sign or high-risk situation management, a relapse prevention network needs to be developed. An effective relapse prevention network consists of the patient, the therapist, family members and/or significant others, healthcare professionals, and appropriate Twelve-Step support people (such as a Pills Anonymous sponsor).

The patient works with this network to develop a relapse intervention plan. This is one more way APM™ patients can take an active role in their recovery process. They share their high-risk situations and warning signs with the network and inform each member of what to do if any active warning signs and/or symptoms of chemical use arise. Identifying early critical warning signs and sharing that knowledge with the relapse prevention network greatly increases the chances of stopping a relapse process before the actual chemical use begins.

> High-risk situations are any experiences that
> activate urges to self-medicate despite
> patients' best intentions not to relapse.

As discussed earlier, relapse prevention counseling starts with assessment and treatment planning followed by a high-risk situation identification process. A high-risk situation is any experience that can activate the urge to use inappropriate pain medication (including alcohol or other drugs) despite the commitment not to. It is a situation that makes a patient want to stop using their effective pain management program despite promises to themselves or others.

The following section explains Exercise Five in the *Addiction-Free Pain Management™ Workbook*, the High-Risk Situation exercise.

- **Exercise Five:**
  Identifying and Personalizing Your High-Risk Situations

Defining the concept of a high-risk situation can be complicated. Some situations activate self-defeating urges for some people and not others. The same situation can activate the urges at some times but not at others. Exercise Five is broken down into three separate parts. Part 1 is designed to help patients identify a high-risk situation they will be facing in the near future and then to personalize it. Patients start doing this by completing the following exercise from the *Addiction-Free Pain Management™ Workbook*.

Exercise Five, Part 1:
Identifying an Immediate Pain and
Medication High-Risk Situation

Defining High-Risk Situations

A high-risk situation is something that happens that creates an urge to use inappropriate pain medication or other drugs (including alcohol) after making a commitment not to. It can also be a situation that creates an urge to stop using your effective pain management program despite your promises to yourself. You don't get into high-rish situations by accident. But sometimes you mistakenly believe that you are drawn to these situations. Once you are in the situation, you don't know what to do. You convince yourself that it's really not your fault that you are in this situation, that you didn't plan it, that it just happened and there's nothing you can do about it. Defining the concept of a high-risk situation can be tricky. The same type of situation can be a problem at one time, but not another.

1. **Identify an immediate high-risk situation:** Think ahead over the next several weeks, and identify a situation that could tempt you to deviate from your Medication Management Agreement despite your commitment not to use inappropriately. Or identify a situation that would cause you to stop working an effective pain management plan. Write a short sentence that describes that situation.

2. **How does this situation increase your risk of using pain medication?** Write one or two sentences that describe how this situation might change your thinking or behavior and lead you to violate your Medication Management Agreement or sabotage your effective pain management.

3. **Write a personal title:** In the space below write a word or short phrase that accurately describes your high-risk situation. This word or phrase should be in your words and have emotional impact on you. Personal Title: _____

4. **Write a personal description:** Write a complete sentence that describes the high-risk situation. Do not use any of the words that you used in your Personal Title and follow this format: *I know I'm in a high-risk situation when <I do something> that causes <pain> and I think about or have an urge to use inap-*

propriate pain medication (including alcohol or other drugs) to manage the pain or to solve my problems. Example: I know I'm in a high-risk situation when <I stop swimming daily> and that causes <my lower back to start hurting> so I start fantasizing about taking my old pills to make my pain go away.

5. **Risk of using inappropriate pain medication:** How high a risk are you for using inappropriate pain medication or other self-defeating behaviors to manage this situation?
(Patients are asked to pick a rating between 0 and 10.)

6. **Why do you rate your risk at that level?** Please explain your answer.

Jean's High-Risk Situation

Jean identified a situation where she was going to have to meet with her oldest daughter's schoolteacher for parent-teacher night. She recognized that this situation increased her stress levels and intensified her pain. She reported feeling a strong sense of shame, because the teacher knew about her medication problems; the school environment also triggered flashbacks from her own school trauma history.

The title she chose was "I can't do this." She completed the sentence this way: "I know I'm in a high-risk situation when I get upset and ashamed, then my stress level goes up, which causes my pain to increase and I want to take a pill." She believed she only had a 50 to 60 percent chance of using her medication inappropriately at this point, because she could not see any other options.

Dean's High-Risk Situation

Dean chose a situation where it was likely he would have to confront his fear of talking about the affair he had. His wife asked him to start couples therapy with the expectation that he would be emotionally open and truthful with her during their sessions.

The title he chose was "pure panic." He reported that he was especially afraid, because if she found out about his past affairs, she would divorce him and he would be all alone. He completed the sentence this way: "I know I'm in a high-risk situation when I tell myself I need to take something to boost my courage and take the edge off my fear." He believed that he rated at a 60 to 70 percent chance of using, so he was very anxious.

Part 2 of Exercise Five in the *Addiction-Free Pain Management™ Workbook* asks patients to read the high-risk situation developed specifically for the APM™ population. The list below contains nineteen common high-risk situations for this population.

Exercise Five, Part 2: Reading the APM High-Risk Situation List

Instructions:

As you read each of the high-risk situations (HRS) below, rate each high-risk situation on a scale of 0 to 10, with 0 meaning this has not, does not, and probably will not apply to me and 10 meaning that it has been, is, or could be a serious problem for me. Realize that you may have an urge to minimize or rationalize these situations, or some people may even start feeling very upset by what they read. If this happens to you, note it so you can share this reaction with someone you trust.

---

1. ❐ **We only want to stop because we have problems:** We experience a serious problem or crisis related to our pain medication (including alcohol) or other drug use. We feel an inner conflict. One part of us wants to keep taking the medication despite the problem. Another part of us says no and holds us back, because going back to using inappropriately would cause even more serious problems. We convince ourselves that it would be a good idea to stop taking the medication until the situation calms down, but we feel deprived. Since we don't believe we can continue coping with life without our pain medication, we leave the door open to change our mind later when things have calmed down.

2. ❐ **We don't see the connection:** We are blind to the relationship between our use of pain medication (including alcohol) or other drugs, and the problems that we're having. We convince ourselves that we need to use pain medication despite the problems. Nobody has the right to make us stop. We tell ourselves that the real problem isn't our pain medi-

cation—it's the pain we have. Sure we've got some serious problems. That's why we're taking the medication—to help us cope with those problems. Besides, a doctor prescribed it for us, so it must be all right.

3. ❐ **We deny we have a problem with medication:** We tell ourselves that we're in control of our pain medication use; it doesn't control us. We can stop forever if only the pain would stop for good. We're not taking the medication now and that proves we're in control. Nobody is going to convince us that we're weak-willed or some kind of a drug addict.

4. ❐ **We push away those who threaten our continued pain medication use:** We prove we're not an addict or drug abuser by telling ourselves that we have friends and people who care about us and they don't see a problem with our using the medication the way we are. There are other people who don't like us using the medication the way we are. It's these people, who aren't really our friends, who want us to stop and even suffer with our pain. If they were really our friends, they wouldn't be causing us problems by sticking their noses in where they don't belong. They would realize that we deserve to have the medication. If they'd just leave us alone, then everything would be just fine.

5. ❐ **We only remember the good times:** We start remembering how good it was to use our pain medication in the past. We make our memories bigger than life by exaggerating the relief we got while minimizing or blocking out the emotional pain and the negative side effects we experienced. We start to convince ourselves that we always felt good and never experienced any pain or problems when we were taking our pain medication the way we wanted.

6. ❐ **We "awfulize" being without pain medication:** We start thinking about how hard it is to stay away from pain medication. We convince ourselves that it is awful, terrible, and unbearable to have to live without using our pain medication the way we want. Sober living is nothing but pain, problems, and hassles. Without pain medication we can never have a pain-free, good quality of life.

7. ❏ **We use magical thinking:** We believe that pain medication can magically fix us. We mistakenly believe that pain medication would always make us feel good and solve all of our problems. We convince ourselves that this time we won't abuse it or lose control. We'll use it responsibly. Besides, it will just be this one time. We'll only use for a short period of time until the pain settles down. Then we'll just stop again.

8. ❏ **We get into problem situations:** We start putting ourselves into situations that create unnecessary stress, pain, and problems. Sometimes we make our pain worse when we have a legitimate pain flare-up by doing things that make it worse instead of better. We shoot ourselves in the foot by not using effective pain management and experience the negative consequences. Then we reload the gun and shoot ourselves in the other foot.

9. ❏ **We overcommit:** Sometimes we take on more than we can handle and start missing deadlines and letting other people down. This causes our stress to increase leading to our pain getting worse. Instead of talking openly about our problems, we go underground, put things off, blame others, and try to cover our tracks. If we get caught, we get defensive and try to rationalize or explain our way out of it.

10. ❏ **We get frustrated:** Sometimes we get frustrated because we want something that we can't have—a totally pain free life. When this happens, we feel deprived because we should be able to have it. We deserve it. We're entitled to it. Others don't have the right to keep us from getting it, even if we need to use inappropriate pain medication to obtain it.

11. ❏ **We want to fit in:** We feel left out. It seems like no one likes us or wants to be around us since our pain condition limits us so much. We want to fit in and feel like a normal person again, but somehow we just can't see ourselves doing that without resorting to using inappropriate pain medication.

12. ❏ **We seek out a pain medication supportive environment:** We start putting ourselves in situations where we're around people, places, and things that make us want to use

inappropriate pain medication despite our commitment not to. We might get into situations where we're feeling good, but we want to feel even better or enjoy ourselves more. We don't know how to without using inappropriate pain medication.

13. ☐ **We want to change our energy:** We might get into situations that stress us out or make us feel tired or bored. These situations leave us feeling like we need something to either calm us down or to pick us up.

14. ☐ **We see people enjoying themselves:** We might be in a social situation. The people we're with are having a very good time and being very active. We suddenly notice that everyone else is doing things that we can't do without taking extra pain medication. We don't want to use pain medication, but everyone else is having so much fun and we feel pressured. We remember how good it could be and ask ourselves, "Why not?" Besides no one will know.

15. ☐ **We want better sex:** We might get into a sexual experience that couldn't happen without using pain medication. Or a sexual experience might not be going as well as we would like because of our pain. We know that pain medication could improve our performance, increase our pleasure, get rid of our limitations, and help us to seduce or please our partner.

16. ☐ **We face a loss:** A family member or friend might die. We have to go to the funeral and attend the social functions that surround it. We see people using alcohol or other drugs to cope with their pain. We know that one relative has tranquilizers and will give them to anyone who wants them. We remember that our old pain medication could help us feel better too. We don't give in but then we go home, alone, to deal with the pain and loss. We want to feel better, but we just don't know what to do without using pain meds.

17. ☐ **We remember the "good old days":** We find ourselves daydreaming about how healthy and active we used to be, or sometimes we wake up from dreaming about participating in our old favorite physical activities. When we realize it is only a dream, we feel cheated and frustrated. We need to grieve

the loss of our healthy self, but we don't know how and instead we become tempted to use inappropriate medication to escape.

18. ☐ **We feel trapped:** We might get into a situation where we feel isolated or cut off from others. We might get backed into a corner and start feeling trapped because we don't know what to do. It seems like there is no way to fit in or get connected. To avoid situations like this, we might start spending more time alone and when we're by ourselves, we might start to feel lonely. When our pain is bad, we don't reach out; we suffer all alone.

19. ☐ **We get sick or injured:** We might get sick, injured, or start having different physical pain or discomfort. A doctor might offer us a prescription for pain medication, muscle relaxants, or tranquilizers. What's wrong with that? He/She is a doctor and we're sick or in pain, which is different than our other condition. We deserve relief. We don't mention our past problems with pain medication.

The next exercise in the *Addiction-Free Pain Management™ Workbook* asks patients to use what they learned by reading the high-risk situation list and modify the high-risk situation they chose in Part 1. See the following exercise.

Exercise Five, Part 3:
Indentifying and Finalizing
Your APM High-Risk Situation

Discussion Questions

1. What is the high-risk situation that you will be facing in the immediate future that could cause you to use inappropriate pain medication (including alcohol) or other drugs despite your commitment not to?

2. What did you learn from reading the APM High-Risk Situation List that can help you better understand and clarify this high-risk situation?

---

3. What was your previous personal title for the high-risk situation? Do you need to modify your personal title after reading the high-risk situation list? Remember that the title should stir up a feeling or emotion. The title should not be any longer than two or three words. An example of a personal title for the sample description below is "Getting Complacent." What is your new personal title for your high-risk situation?

Personal Title: _____

4. See if you need to revise your personal description for the high-risk situation that you selected. The description should start with the words "I know that I'm in a high-risk situation when I...." You should use something that you learned by reading the high-risk situation list to make the description even more concrete and specific. Remember to use the general format below:

I know that I am in a high-risk situation when *<I do something or get involved in something>* that causes *<pain and problems>* and I want to use inappropriate pain medication (including alcohol) or other drugs to manage the pain and solve the problems. **Example:** I know that I am in a high-risk situation when *<I stop swimming daily>* and that causes *<my back to start hurting more>* so I want to take a pill to make my pain go away.

Jean's Magical Thinking

Jean identified with the magical thinking high-risk situation. **We use magical thinking**: *We believe that pain medication can magically fix us. We mistakenly believe that pain medication will always make us feel good and solve all of our problems. We convince ourselves that this time we won't abuse it or lose control. We'll use it responsibly. Besides, it will just be this one time. We'll only use for a short period of time until the pain settles down. Then we'll just stop again.*

She realized she was using the added stress and shame as an excuse to use pain medication to help her deal with an uncomfortable situation—the way she used to do it. She changed her title to "I'm doing it again." She changed her programming sentence this way: "I know I'm in a high-risk situation when I start fantasizing about how well my medication used to help me escape my feelings, and

I begin to self-destruct by convincing myself I have a right to use any way I want."

> Dean is feeling trapped.

Dean chose the situation pertaining to fear. **We feel trapped:** *We might get into a situation where we feel isolated or cut off from others. We might get backed into a corner and start feeling trapped because we don't know what to do. It seems like there is no way to fit in or get connected. To avoid situations like this, we might start spending more time alone, and when we're by ourselves, we might start to feel lonely. When our pain is bad, we don't reach out; we suffer all alone.*

Dean realized that past situations like this led him to isolate and escape. He decided to change his title from "Pure panic" to "Run and hide." He decided his programming sentence was good the way it was: "I know I'm in a high-risk situation when I tell myself I need to take something to boost my courage and take the edge off my fear." Dean's extramarital affairs were very serious issues, but now was not the time to attempt resolution, so the process of "Bookmarking" was used. However, Dean did agree that he needed to immediately learn how to face the situation of being more emotionally present and open with his wife.

> Using a *Bookmarking* Interviewing Skill

Bookmarking is an interviewing skill that allows patients to identify and clarify secondary issues and problems as they emerge, explore the relationship of those issues to the current target problem, write it down, and agree to work on it later in recovery. See the bookmarking process in the following table.

The Bookmarking Process

- Allow the patient to briefly explain their problem or issue.
- Use active listening to show the patient he or she is listened to, understood, and taken seriously.
- Write down the issue on a card or sheet of paper. Have the patient write the issue down in his or her workbook. Many clinicians have a section in their notes for bookmarked issues.
- Explain to the patient that this issue is important.
- Ask the patient what would happen to their ability to resolve this issue if they started to use inappropriate medication again, including alcohol or other drugs.
- Remind the patient of the tasks that you are trying to complete, and assure them that you will return to the bookmarked issues as soon as appropriate.

Working on a charged issue too soon, such as Dean's history of extramarital affairs, could very well lead to a relapse. It was in Dean's best interest to avoid *brutal honesty* at this point in his recovery process.

Using Exercise Six, Situation Mapping, as an appropriate intervention to teach Dean how to deal with the immediate high-risk situation in a safe way, allowed him to focus first on how to be open and present with his wife. Dean also talked with his sponsor about not rushing in with a *true confession* until his recovery was more stable. His sponsor reminded him that he was only on Step 3 of his Twelve-Step program, and *Making Amends* was in Step 9. He had some time before it would be necessary to deal with his extramarital affairs.

• Exercise Six: Situation Mapping

Exercise Six is divided into three parts. Part 1 asks patients to think of a specific time when they experienced their high-risk situation and coped with it in a way that caused them to use inappropriate pain medication or other drugs (including alcohol) and/or used ineffective pain management. Patients are asked to think about the experience as if it were a story with a beginning, middle, and end.

Part 2 asks patients to think of a specific time when they experienced this high-risk situation and managed it using effective pain management, and/or avoided using inappropriate pain medication or other drugs (including alcohol). Unfortunately, many patients have no experience of coping with high-risk situations without using medication inappropriately or other self-defeating behaviors. When this is the case, ask the patient, "What would it be like to manage such a situation effectively?"

In Part 3 patients are asked to think of the most important high-risk situation they will be experiencing in the near future. They are asked to imagine themselves using ineffective pain management or other self-defeating behaviors that would cause them to use inappropriate pain medication or other drugs (including alcohol). They are asked to imagine themselves doing the things they would have done in the past to convince themselves it is justifiable to use inappropriate pain medication or other drugs (including alcohol).

Both Jean and Dean were able to identify appropriate mapping situations that brought them more clarity about past using incidents. By answering the remaining questions in the mapping processes, both patients were able to identify three intervention points where they could have done something different to change the outcome. The remainder of the questions for the mapping processes follows.

Exercise Six, Parts 1, 2, and 3: Discussion Questions

2. What did you want to accomplish by managing this situation the way you did?

3. Did you get what you wanted by managing the situation this way?

   ❏ Yes ❏ No ❏ Unsure

   Explain:_____

   _____

   _____

4. On a scale of 1 to 10, what were your stress levels when you managed the situation this way? _____

5. On a scale of 1 to 10, what were your pain levels when you managed the situation this way? _____

6. **Doing something different:** Can you think of some things that you could have done differently to manage the situation

---

215

without having to use inappropriate pain medication (including alcohol) or other drugs or other self-defeating behaviors?

7. **Avoiding the situation:** What could you have done to responsibly avoid getting into this situation?

   If you avoided this situation, how would it have changed the outcome?

8. **Decision point #1:** What could you have done differently near the beginning of the situation to produce a better outcome? (How could you have thought differently? managed your feelings and emotions differently? responded to your self-destructive urges differently? acted or behaved differently? treated other people differently?)

   If you did these things, how would it change the situation?

9. **Decision point #2:** What could you have done differently near the middle of the situation to produce a better outcome? (How could you have thought differently? managed your feelings and emotions differently? responded to your self-destructive urges differently? acted or behaved differently? treated other people differently?)

   If you did these things, how would it change the outcome?

10. **Decision point #3:** What you have done differenly near the end of the situation to produce a better outcome? (How could you have thought differently? managed your feelings and emotions differently? responded to your self-destructive urges differently? acted or behaved differently? treated other people differently?)

    If you did these things, how would it change the outcome?

11. **Stop relapse quickly:** If you start using inappropriate pain medication (including alcohol) or other drugs, what can you do to stop?

12. **Most important thing learned:** What is the most important thing that you learned by completing this exercise?

    Note: If you do relapse, it is important not to despair. You can choose to learn from that situation and discover that in the future you will be able to intervene before you use inappropriately or experience life-damaging consequences. The important thing is that you learn to intervene as soon as you are able. For some people the recovery process seems to move steadily forward, but for many others it goes forward, the person hits a stuck point, consolidates their resources, and then moves forward again. Whatever your recovery pattern is, you must not give up. Remember, recovery is a lifelong learning process.

Up to now most of this work has been to help patients uncover and understand the problems associated with the *Addiction Pain Syndrome*. In the next chapter you will learn how Jean and Dean discovered ways to further understand and manage their high-risk situations. This is accomplished through the use of the *TFUAR Process*.

• **Call to Action for the Eighth Chapter**

It is time to summarize what you learned now that you have come to the end of the eighth chapter. Please answer the questions below.

1.   What is the most important thing you learned about yourself and your ability to help addicted pain patients as a result of completing Chapter Eight?

2.   What are you willing to commit to do differently as a result of what you have learned by completing this chapter?

3.   What obstacles might get in the way of making these changes? What can you do to overcome these roadblocks?

Take time to pause and reflect, then go to the next page to review Chapter Nine.

Chapter Nine

The TFUAR Process and Recovery Planning

- **Exercise Seven: Analyzing and Managing High-Risk Situations**

Exercise Seven in the *Addiction-Free Pain Management™ Workbook* is focused on analyzing and managing high-risk situations using the TFUAR Process. As mentioned earlier, TFUAR stands for thinking, feelings, urges, actions, and reactions or relationships.

TFUAR Process
• Thoughts (T) cause feelings (F)
• Thoughts plus feelings cause urges (U)
• Urges plus decisions cause actions (A)
• Actions cause social reactions (R)
• Two types of TFUAR sequences:
—Self-defeating
—Addictive

In this exercise patients learn how to analyze their high-risk situation by identifying the thoughts, feelings, urges, actions, and reactions of others that are related to coping with the high-risk situation in a way that leads to relapse. Once they analyze their problematic or addictive TFUARs, they have an opportunity to start developing new recovery-prone ways to manage their TFUARs.

Some patients may have difficulty separating their TFUARs. They might not be able to distinguish thoughts from feelings. They may not believe the way they think has any effect on their feelings. They may not be able to distinguish feelings from urges or recognize that each feeling carries with it a specific urge. They may not realize they can experience a feeling—sit still and breathe through it until it dissipates without acting upon it. They may not be able to recognize the space between an urge and an action.

Impulse control lives in that space between the urge and the action. Patients can be taught to expand this in-between space so that they pause and notice the urge, but do nothing about it. From a place of *reflection,* patients can begin to question themselves: *What do I have an urge to do*? What has happened when I have done similar things in the past? What is likely to happen if I do that now? They can now make an appropriate decision: *What do I choose to do*? I know I will be responsible for the action and its consequences.

Some patients may not be able to distinguish action from social reaction. They may believe that people are reacting to them for no reason at all. They may not link the responses of others to their own behaviors.

The following flow chart shows the progression from the high-risk situation trigger all the way to the social reaction. You will also see an item labeled *positive self-talk*—the starting point for moving out of the problem and into the solution. The chart shows some areas that patients can interject this way of thinking in order to have a more positive outcome. As you can see, the last place positive self-talk can help change the outcome is at the decision point. Relapse prevention means teaching patients a concept called *time-line competency*—learning from the past then taking that knowledge into the present to plan for the future.

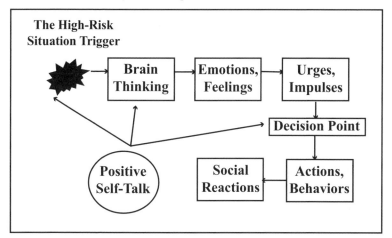

With the above information in mind, let's look at Exercise Seven in the *Addiction-Free Pain Management™ Workbook*, which has six parts. Part 1 asks patients to think of a high-risk situation they are working on and then analyze their TFUARs. On the following pages you will find this six-part workbook exercise.

Exercise Seven, Part 1:
Looking at Your Personal Reactions
to High-Risk Situations

High-risk situations, such as the ones you mapped out in the previous exercise, can activate deeply entrenched habits of thinking, feeling, acting, and relating to others that create an urge to abuse your pain medication or stop your effective pain management practices. To effectively manage these high-risk situations, you must learn to understand and control the way you react in these situations. Your chances of managing high-risk situations without using pain medication, including alcohol or other drugs, go up as you get better at recognizing and managing your thoughts, feelings, urges, actions, and social reactions that create the urge to deviate from your medication management agreement.

Let's define some words that will help you understand the process of learning how to manage your reactions to high-risk situations.

Personal reactions are automatic habitual things that you do when situations occur. There are four things that automatically take place when these situations come up: You think about it, you have feelings or emotional reactions to it, you get an urge to do something about it, and you actually do something about it. So each automatic personal reaction can be broken down into its component parts, which are: (1) automatic thoughts, (2) automatic feelings, (3) automatic urges, and (4) automatic actions. To learn how to effectively manage high-risk situations, you must learn to change automatic reactions into conscious choices.

Personal responses are different from personal reactions. A personal reaction is automatic and unconscious. A response is something you consciously choose to do. A conscious response is a choice. In order to manage high-risk situations without using pain medication, including alcohol or other drugs, you must learn to make better choices about how to respond to situations. In other words, to change automatic responses into conscious choices, you must choose what you think, how you manage and express your feelings, how you manage your urges, and what you actually do in these situations.

Addictive thinking is an irrational way of thinking that convinces you that using inappropriate pain medication, including alcohol and other drugs, is an effective way to manage the pain and problems caused by irresponsible thinking and behavior.

Irresponsible thinking is an irrational way of thinking about something that causes unnecessary emotional pain and motivates you to do things that will make your problems worse.

Addictive behavior is a way of acting that puts you around people, places, and things that make you want to use inappropriate pain medication, including alcohol or other drugs.

Irresponsible behavior is a way of acting out or behaving that causes unnecessary pain and problems.

There are **emotional consequences** to thoughts and actions. All thoughts and behaviors have logical consequences. Sober, responsible, or rational thinking allows you to deal with life without experiencing unnecessary emotional pain or the urge to use inappropriate pain medication, including alcohol or other drugs, to manage unpleasant feelings. Sober and responsible behavior allows you to conduct your life and solve your problems without producing unnecessary complications for yourself or others and without having to center your life around the inappropriate use of pain medication, including alcohol or other drugs.

Instant Gratification is the desire to feel better now even if it means you will hurt worse in the future. When you seek instant gratification, you want to do something, anything that will instantly make you feel better. **You want to feel better now without having to think better or act better first. This results in a quick-fix mentality.** When you seek instant gratification, you want to feel good all of the time. You tend to place "feeling good" above all other priorities. This is often based on the mistaken belief that "If I feel better, I will be better and my life will be better!" You are not interested in living according to a responsible set of principles that will make your life work well. You want what you want when you want it regardless of the consequences.

Deferred Gratification is the ability to feel uncomfortable or to hurt now in order to gain a benefit or to feel better in the future. When you use deferred gratification, you think and act better first in order to feel better later. To learn how to develop deferred gratification you must get in the habit of *thinking things through before you act them out*. Deferred gratification is based on the belief that there are rules or principles that will make your life work well in the long run and will give you a firm sense of meaning, purpose, and satisfaction that will allow you to get through the inevitable periods of pain, hard feelings, and frustration that are a normal part of life and living.

You can learn how to *challenge addictive and irresponsible thoughts*. You must learn how to identify and challenge your addictive and irresponsible thoughts if you want to make responsible choices that will allow you to build an effective and satisfying way of life. The following way of thinking can help you challenge the tendency to seek instant gratification. The healthy goal is to live a good life regardless of how it feels at the moment. Feelings change, effective principles don't. Sober and responsible people live a life based on principles, not feelings. Instant gratification provides what looks like an easy way out. The problem is that this easy way out becomes a trap. Once trapped in a conditioned pattern of instant gratification, you will feel cravings when you attempt to break the pattern. But once the pattern is broken, the urges disappear because the long-term beneficial consequences of responsible living kick in.

In the following exercise on *Managing Personal Reaction to High-Risk Situations*, you will learn how to analyze your high-risk situations by identifying the thoughts, feelings, urges, actions, and social reactions that make you want to deviate from your medication management agreement. Then you will learn how to manage them in a new and more effective way without using inappropriate pain medication, including alcohol or other drugs.

1. *Thoughts cause feelings.* Whenever you think about something, you automatically react by having a feeling or an emotion.

2. *Thoughts and feelings work together to cause urges.* Your way of thinking causes you to feel certain feelings. These feelings, in turn, reinforce the way you are thinking. These thoughts and feelings work together to create an urge to do something. An urge is a desire that may be rational or irrational. The irrational urge to use inappropriate pain medication, including alcohol or other drugs, even though you know it will hurt you, is also called *craving*. It is irrational because you want to use even though you know it will not be good for you.

3. *Urges plus decisions cause actions.* A decision is a choice. A choice is a specific way of thinking that causes you to commit to one way of doing things while refusing to do anything else. The space between the urge and the action is filled with a decision. This decision may be an automatic and unconscious choice that you have learned to make without having to think about it, or this decision can be based on a conscious choice

that results from carefully reflecting on the situation and the options available for dealing with it.

4. *Actions cause reactions from other people.* Your actions affect other people and cause them to react to you. It is helpful to think about your behavior like invitations that you give to other people to treat you in certain ways. Some behaviors invite people to be nice to you and to treat you with respect. Other behaviors invite people to argue and fight with you or to put you down. In every social situation you share a part of the responsibility for what happens, because you are constantly inviting people to respond to you by the actions you take and how you react to what other people do.

Relapse usually involves one or more of the following problems:

1. *You can't tell the difference between thoughts and feelings.* You also tend to believe you can think anything that you want and it won't affect your feelings. Then when you start to feel bad you can't understand why and convince yourself the only way to feel better is to use pain medication, including alcohol or other drugs.

2. *You can't tell the difference between feelings and urges.* You believe each feeling carries with it a specific urge. You don't realize you can experience a feeling: sit still and breathe into the feeling and it will go away without being acted on.

3. *You can't tell the difference between urges and actions.* You don't realize there is a space between urge and action—the decision point.

4. *You can't control your impulses.* You believe you must do whatever you feel an urge to do. You have never understood that to learn impulse control you must learn how to pause, relax, reflect, and decide even when you feel a strong urge to act immediately. The following are four steps in the impulse control process:

    • *Pause* and notice the urge without doing anything about it.

    • *Relax* by taking a deep breath, slowly exhaling, and consciously imagining the stress draining from your body.

    • *Reflect* on what you are experiencing by asking yourself, "What do I have an urge to do? What has happened when I have done similar things in the past? What is likely to happen if I do that now?"

- *Decide* what you are going to do about the urge. Make a conscious choice instead of acting out in an automatic and unconscious way. When making the choice about what you are going to do, remind yourself that you will be responsible for both the action that you choose to take and its consequence.

Remember: *Impulse control lives in the space between the urge and the action.*

5. *You can't tell the difference between actions and social reactions.* You tend to believe that people respond to you for no reason at all. You don't link the responses of others to what you do when you are with others. In reality what you do gives an invitation to other people to treat you in certain ways. Ask yourself: "How do I want to invite other people to treat me in this situation?"

    With this in mind, the following exercise will help you identify and change the thoughts, feelings, urges, actions, and social reactions that can lead you back to using pain medication, including alcohol and other drugs.

Part 1 of this exercise is meant to be an educational component that helps patients understand what they are going to be doing and why it is so important. Like most of the patients I worked with, Dean and Jean were able to complete the following exercises much more effectively after reading and discussing this information. Sometimes information needs to be simplified for patients. It is imperative that the healthcare provider not only understands, but internalizes this information so they can articulate it in such a way that the patient fully comprehends it.

Exercise Seven, Part 2:
Managing Thoughts That Cause You to Use Inappropriate Medication

In order to manage high-risk situations, you must learn to identify the thoughts that can create an urge to use inappropriate pain medication, including alcohol and other drugs, and/or indulge in other self-defeating behaviors. Think of a high-risk situation that you want to learn how to manage more effectively.

---

1. Go back to the exercise, *Identifying and Personalizing Your High-Risk Situations*, and write the title and description of the high-risk situation that you will be facing in the near future in the spaces below:

Title of Your High-Risk Situation:

Description of the High-Risk Situation: *I know that I'm in a high-risk situation when I...*

2. Keeping the situation you described above in mind, read each of the thoughts listed below. Ask yourself if you tend to think similar thoughts when you are in this high-risk situation. If you do, put a check in the box in front of the thought. Check as many boxes as you need to.

☐ 1. I don't have a serious pain medication problem, so there is no good reason for me not to use pain medication to deal with this situation.

☐ 2. I have a right to use pain medication in this situation, and nobody has the right to tell me to stop.

☐ 3. If I use pain medication to deal with this situation, nobody will know about it. So what difference will it make?

☐ 4. If I use pain medication to deal with this situation, nothing bad will happen to me as a result.

☐ 5. If I don't use pain medication, I won't be able to effectively manage this situation.

☐ 6. If I don't use pain medication, I won't be able to handle the stress and pain that this situation will cause.

☐ 7. Pain medication can help me manage this situation more effectively.

☐ 8. I shouldn't have to do anything special to manage this situation. If I just go with the flow, everything will be OK.

3. What are the three thoughts you tend to have in this kind of high-risk situation that makes you want to use pain medication? You can use the thoughts above as a starting point, but it is important for you to write down these thoughts in your own words.

Part 2 asks the patient to think of the high-risk situation they want to learn how to manage effectively without using inappropriate pain medication and/or other drugs (including alcohol). They are asked to read each of the addictive thoughts and ask themselves if they think similar thoughts when they are in the high-risk situation. If they do, they are to check the box in front of the thought(s) they picked, put the thoughts in their own words, and then come up with a challenge for each one.

Jean's Addictive Thought Selections

In this exercise Jean picked numbers 2, 4, and 5. This exercise helped her see previously unconscious thoughts that led to the inappropriate use of her pain medication. She especially focused on item 2 because she realized this was connected to one of her major denial patterns called: *I have the right to be this way; AKA it's my body.* Jean also realized she needed help in dismantling her magical thinking in 4 and 5 regarding her minimization and rationalization about what would happen if she used. She was excited to start learning more effective thinking management skills.

Jean put her three major self-defeating thoughts in her own words. "They don't know what it's like, so they should just get off my case." Other thoughts she had were: "It won't get out of control this time" and "I'll freak if I don't use." It took Jean a long time to come up with effective challenging interventions for those thoughts. Her top three were: (1) "People are concerned—I should listen"; (2) "I know better—it will get out of control"; and (3) "I have new tools now—I'll be OK." She realized this was just a starting point and looked forward to the remainder of the exercise.

Dean's Addictive Thought Selections

Dean chose items 2, 3, and 7, but he also stated that some of the others could apply to him as well. Dean was surprised at how many of these thoughts he actually experienced when he was in high-risk situations. His special focus item was number 3. This was related to his major isolation pattern as well as the way he avoided being totally honest with anyone—especially his wife.

Dean realized that this pattern of convincing himself "it was necessary to keep secrets" was connected to one of his major denial patterns called *Rationalizing.* Like Jean, he also saw that he used another favorite denial pattern, *I have the right to be this way; AKA it's my body,* to justify his continued use of self-defeating behaviors, including isolation and inappropriate medication use so he could avoid feeling uncomfortable emotions.

Dean put his three major self-defeating thoughts in his own words. "Screw them! I'm the one in pain here." His other self-defeating thoughts were: "They'll never know" and "Using will get me through this." It took Dean a long time and much frustration before he was able to come up with effective challenging interventions for those thoughts. His top three were: (1) "They really want to help me—I'll let them"; (2) "Keeping secrets hurts me and those I love"; and (3) "I can do this without using." He saw that painful emotions, especially guilt and shame, were a problem area and looked forward to learning new feeling management skills.

Exercise Seven, Part 3:
Managing Feelings That Cause You to Use Inappropriate Medication

The following exercise will show you how to more effectively manage the feelings and emotions that you will tend to experience in your immediate high-risk situation:

1. Before completing this part of the exercise, go back and read the title and description of the high-risk situation that you are learning how to manage.

2. When you are in this high-risk situation, do you tend to feel...
   ❐ Strong?   or   ❐ Weak?
   How intense is the feeling? (0–10) _____
   Why do you rate it this way?

3. When you are in this high-risk situation, do you tend to feel...
   ❐ Angry?   or   ❐ Caring?
   How intense is the feeling? (0–10) _____
   Why do you rate it this way?

4. When you are in this high-risk situation, do you tend to feel...
   ❐ Happy?   or   ❐ Sad?
   How intense is the feeling? (0–10) _____
   Why do you rate it this way?

5. When you are in this high-risk situation, do you tend to feel...
   ❐ Safe?   or   ❐ Threatened?
   How intense is the feeling? (0–10) _____
   Why do you rate it this way?

6. When you are in this high-risk situation, do you tend to feel…

   ❏ Fulfilled?   or   ❏ Frustrated?
   How intense is the feeling? (0–10) _____
   Why do you rate it this way?

7. When you are in this high-risk situation, do you tend to feel…

   ❏ Proud?   or   ❏ Ashamed?
   How intense is the feeling? (0–10) _____
   Why do you rate it this way?

8. When you are in this high-risk situation, do you tend to feel…

   ❏ Lonely?   or   ❏ Connected?
   How intense is the feeling? (0–10) _____
   Why do you rate it this way?

9. When you are in this high-risk situation, do you tend to feel…

   ❏ Peaceful?   or   ❏ Agitated?
   How intense is the feeling? (0–10) _____
   Why do you rate it this way?

10. What are the three strongest feelings you tend to have in this kind of high-risk situation that makes you want to use inappropriate pain medication, including alcohol or other drugs?

11. Keeping these three feelings in mind, read each of the following statements about your ability to manage your feelings, and rate how true it is on a scale of 0–10 (0 means the statement is not at all true. 10 means the statement is totally true.) Place your answer on the line in front of each statement.

___ A. **Skill #1:** I am able to anticipate situations that are likely to provoke strong feelings and emotions.

___ B. **Skill #2:** I am able to recognize when I am starting to have a strong feeling or emotion.

___ C. **Skill #3:** I am able to stop myself from automatically reacting to the feeling without thinking it through.

___ D. **Skill #4:** I am able to call a time-out in emotionally-charged situations before my feelings become unmanageable.

___ E. **Skill #5:** I am able to use an immediate relaxation technique to bring down the intensity of the feeling.

___ F. **Skill #6:** I am able to take a deep breath and notice what I'm feeling.

___ G. **Skill #7:** I am able to find words that describe what I'm feeling and use the feeling list when necessary.

____ H. **Skill #8:** I am able to rate the intensity of my feelings using a ten-point scale.

____ I. **Skill #9:** I am able to consciously acknowledge the feeling and its intensity by saying to myself, "Right now I'm feeling _____ and it's OK to be feeling this way."

____ J. **Skill #10:** I am able to identify what I'm thinking that's making me feel this way and ask myself, "How can I change my thinking in a way that will make me feel better?"

____ K. **Skill #11:** I am able to identify what I'm doing that's making me feel this way and ask myself, "How can I change what I'm doing in a way that will make me feel better?"

____ L. **Skill #12:** I am able to recognize and resist urges to create problems, hurt myself, or hurt other people in an attempt to make myself feel better.

____ M. **Skill #13:** I am able to recognize my resistance to doing things that would help me or my situation and force myself to do those things despite the resistance.

____ N. **Skill #14:** I am able to get outside of myself and recognize and respond to what other people are feeling.

- Select two or three of these feeling management skills that you are willing to commit to getting better at, and list them below.

- Who can you ask to help you with these skills? What could stop you from following through?

- What are any potential obstacles that could keep you from learning these new feeling management skills?

- What are some ways you can overcome any potential obstacles from learning these new feeling management skills?

Part 3 uses the same feeling checklist that was previously covered in an earlier chapter. This time both Jean and Dean saw some differences.

The feelings Jean and Dean chose in Exercise One: Part 3 were: *weak, angry, sad, lonely, threatened,* and *frustrated.* Jean rated *weak* at level 10, while Dean rated it at level 5. Jean rated *sad* at level 8 and Dean rated it at 4. Both rated *anger* and *frustration* at a level 10. Jean rated *ashamed* at level 10, while Dean did not rate either *proud* or *ashamed.* This time Dean was able to see that

229

ashamed was near level 10, and his *sad* rating moved up to level 8. Both rated *lonely* at level 10 this time.

Both Jean and Dean were very happy to work on the "Feeling Management Skills" part of this exercise as they began to learn how they could better manage their uncomfortable feelings.

The instructions for this exercise require the patient to read each statement and rate how true it is for them on a scale of 0–10: 0 means the statement is not at all true and 10 means the statement is totally true. They are then asked to pick two or three of the tools they would like to focus on.

> Learning Feeling Management Skills

Jean noted that before she started the APM™ treatment she would not have been able to have any items near level 10, but now she had three at level 10—items 1, 5, and 8.

Dean had a similar reaction to this exercise. In the past he tended to be a victim of his feelings and would often use pain medication to cope with his uncomfortable emotions. The three most important management skills for him were items 3, 12, and 14. Number 14, *seeking help to deal with feelings*, was a major step forward in Dean's recovery. Although this checklist worked well for Dean and Jean, many patients need additional help to identify and/or articulate their uncomfortable emotions. One tool might be a *Feeling Faces* poster (*http://www.ctherapy.com/feelings_home.asp*) or feeling faces cards (*http://www.feelingfacescards.com/*). These products are commonly used in many treatment programs.

Exercise Seven, Part 4:

Managing Urges That Cause You to Use Inappropriate Medication

High-risk situations often cause the urge to use pain medication, including alcohol and other drugs, or engage in other self-defeating behaviors. When this urge or craving is activated, you almost always experience an inner conflict between two parts of yourself. One part, your addictive self, wants you to use chemicals. Another part of you, the sober self, wants you to manage the situation without using chemicals. This exercise will help you explore these two parts of yourself.

---

1. Before completing this part of the exercise, go back and read the title and the description of the high-risk situation you are learning how to manage.

2. When you are in this high-risk situation, what self-defeating urges do you have?

3. Is there a part of you that wants to use pain medication, including alcohol and drugs? Tell about that part of you.

4. Is there another part of you that wants to manage the situation without using pain medication, including alcohol or drugs? Tell about that part of you.

5. If you wanted to manage this high-risk situation more effectively, what part of you do you need to listen to and why?

Using the Inner Dialogue Process

At this point in the process I find it helpful to use a clinical tool called the *Inner Dialogue Process.* This process is an interviewing skill that is used to help patients identify and clarify the components of internal dissonance. Most patients have an inner conflict between

- the *irresponsible self,* the part of them that believes that the use of irresponsible coping behaviors is good for them, and
- the *responsible self,* the part of them that recognizes the problems with irresponsible coping behaviors.

This inner dialogue technique asks a patient to identify the battle between these two sides of their personality and to learn how to engage in conscious dialogue and train the responsible self to win the arguments. The Inner Dialogue Process includes the following steps:

The Inner Dialogue Process

1. You need to pay careful attention to signs that the patient may be experiencing an inner conflict.

2. When the patient seems conflicted but hasn't said anything, pause and ask, "What's happening? There seems to be a conflict going on inside of you. Is there? Tell me about it."

3. If the patient is strongly asserting one position that supports continued inappropriate coping behavior, ask them, "How

---

strongly do you believe that? Rate your belief on a scale of 1–10, 1 being not very strong and 10 being as strong as you can get." If they say 10, ask them, "Are you sure? Is it possible that there's a small part inside of you that thinks you might be wrong? Can I talk to that part of you for a moment?"

4. The goal is to get the patient to identify both sides of the argument. Then you ask them, "Which side of this argument represents your *irresponsible self*? Why do you think so? Which part of this argument represents your *responsible self*? Why do you think so?"

5. Invite the patients to have the two parts of themselves engage in a conversation by asking, "What would your *irresponsible self* say about this?" Then ask, "What would your *responsible self* say about this?"

This process worked very well for both Jean and Dean. Jean discovered there was a responsible part of her that wanted to quit reacting to her self-defeating urges in ways that hurt her and those she loved. She rated the part that wanted to use medication inappropriately as being very strong—level 7–8 on a 0–10 scale. She was surprised to find she enjoyed talking back to her irresponsible self and realized she did have choices. Dean's process was very similar.

Exercise Seven, Part 5:
Managing Actions That Cause You to Use Inappropriate Medication

1. Before completing this part of the exercise, go back and read the title and the description of the high-risk situation you are learning how to manage.

2. Keeping this high-risk situation in mind, read the following list of self-defeating behaviors that can be used to mismanage this high-risk situation. Check the behaviors you are most likely to use in this situation.

☐ 1. **Proscrastinating:** I put off dealing with the high-risk situation by finding excuses or reasons for not doing it now.

☐ 2. **Distracting myself:** I get too busy with other things to pay attention to managing the situation.

☐ 3. **Saying "It's not important":** I convince myself that other things are more important than effectively managing this high-risk situation.

☐ 4. **Thinking I'm cured:** I convince myself that because I'm OK now and don't have a pain medication problem, there is no need to learn how to manage this high-risk situation.

☐ 5. **Playing dumb:** Even though a big part of me knows what I need to do to manage this situation more effectively, I let myself get confused and convince myself that I can't understand what I'm supposed to do.

☐ 6. **Getting overwhelmed:** I feel scared and start to panic. I use my fear as an excuse for not learning how to manage the high-risk situation more effectively.

☐ 7. **Playing helpless:** I pretend to be too weak and helpless to manage the situation more effectively.

☐ 8. **Wanting the quick fix:** I want a guarantee that I can quickly and easily learn to manage the high-risk situation more effectively or I won't even try.

3. What are the three self-defeating behaviors you tend to have in this kind of high-risk situation that make you want to use pain medication, including alcohol or other drugs? You can use the self-defeating behaviors above as a starting point, but it is important for you to write the descriptions in your own words.

Exercise Seven, Part 5 is about identifying addictive and/or self-defeating tactics that patients have used in the past. In this exercise patients are asked to read the list of *self-defeating behavioral tactics* they can learn to identify and manage in order to creatively implement interactions that will improve their pain management and recovery. They are asked to check the tactic(s) they have used in the past and then list three self-defeating behaviors they have used in past high-risk situations. In addition to identifying the three behaviors, the patient is asked to identify a more recovery-prone way of acting in those types of high-risk situations.

This exercise is an effective tool for helping patients uncover previously automatic and unconscious scripts they have played out over and over again in the past. The first step toward change is recognition that a problem exists. Clinicians familiar with Transactional Analysis (TA) may find some of the above strategies very familiar. Some of the TA tools can be extremely effective in working with recovering people.

> Jean and Dean learned to identify
> and overcome self-defeating behaviors.

When Jean and Dean saw some of the tactics they have used in front of them on the paper, they began to realize how damaging and self-defeating those behaviors were to their recovery process. Jean's most significant realization was noticing a pattern she played out when getting to item 7—"playing helpless." She looked at several of her past significant relationships and saw how she mistakenly believed she could not handle her own situation and asked inappropriate people for help—then she could justify using when they let her down.

Dean's most important awareness was item 8—"wanting the quick fix" or instant gratification. He was able to identify times in the past where he could have avoided using if he would have stuck to his pain management plan, but he stated, "I want it now." The process of analyzing and learning to manage high-risk situations is yet another tool to assist the APM™ patient to move from experiencing themselves as a victim to discovering their own sense of empowerment.

> Tying It All Together

Exercise Seven, Part 6:
Managing Your Personal Reactions
to High-Risk Situations

This exercise will help you tie together everything you have learned by completing the previous management exercises.

1. Before completing this part of the exercise, go back and read the title and the description of the high-risk situation you are learning how to manage. Then review your answers to all of the questions in the previous exercises. Take time to reflect on what you are really saying in your answers. See if you can sense how the answer to each question is somehow connected to all of your other answers. Then complete the following questions:

2. When you are in this high-risk situation, what do you tend to think?	2-a. What is another way of thinking that will allow you to manage this high-risk situation without inappropriately using pain medication?
3. When you're in this high-risk situation, how do you tend to feel?	3-a. What is another way to manage those feelings that will let you manage this situation without inappropriately using pain medication?
4. When you're in this high-risk situation, what do you have a self-defeating urge to do?	4-a. What is another way of managing this urge that will allow you to manage the situation without inappropriately using pain medication?
5. When you're in this high-risk situation, what self-defeating actions do you usually do?	5-a. What are some other things that you could do that will allow you to manage this situation without inappropriately using pain medication?
6. When you're in this high-risk situation, how do other people usually react in ways that cause you distress?	6-a. How could you invite other people to react to you in a way that would help you manage this situation without inappropriately using pain medication?

7. **Most Important Thing Learned:** What is the most important thing you learned by completing this exercise?

8. **Doing Something Different:** What are you going to do differently using what you learned in this exercise?

Jean and Dean experienced some confusion working on the above exercises but eventually worked through their stuck points. Once they realized they had already processed this exercise in the previous worksheets, they became excited. When they finished putting all their answers in the Part 6 table, they had a much better picture of how to more effectively manage any future high-risk situations. To get the greatest benefit from these workbook exercises it is important for patients to work with a professional who has been trained in the CENAPS® Model.

> Treatment works best when patients
> become more proactive in their healing.

- **Exercise Eight: Recovery Planning**

The last clinical exercise in the *Addiction-Free Pain Management™ Workbook* is focused on recovery planning. Having insight and understanding is only the starting point for successful relapse prevention. Developing an effective recovery plan and following it makes the difference between treatment success and failure for most APM™ patients. At this point I often share a phrase I learned from Mr. Gorski: "Insight without action is the booby prize." Dean and Jean thought that was a great way to frame the importance of continuing to be proactive and take action.

> "Insight without action
> is the booby prize."—T. Gorski

While the remainder of this chapter explains recovery planning, the next chapter describes measuring treatment effectiveness. Exercise Eight in the *Addiction-Free Pain Management™ Workbook* assists patients to develop and then test their recovery plan.

Having a structured daily plan assists patients in their recovery process and helps them to practice more effective pain management. The recovery activities suggested in Exercise Eight, Part 1 are a combination of clinical and Twelve-Step activities, along with revisiting many of the nonpharmacological interventions. These recovery principles are proven by the outcome studies from hundreds of chemical dependency treatment centers across the United States and by the successful recovery of millions of people working Twelve-Step recovery programs around the world.

> Effective pain management requires a
> recovery and pain management plan.

Along the same lines, people who are most effective with their pain management have learned to develop a recovery/management plan. However, it is important to note that this plan needs to be individualized to obtain maximum efficiency. Building a personalized recovery, pain management, and relapse prevention plan is essential for optimal treatment success. Many times additional motivational counseling is needed to assist patients in seeing why all this planning is necessary and how it will pay off for them in the long run.

Referring to the following *Addiction Pain Syndrome Diagram,* which was first introduced in Chapter One, a relapse prevention plan must address all three zones concurrently: *the Addictive Disorder Zone, the Pain Disorder Zone,* and *the Addiction Pain Syndrome Zone.*

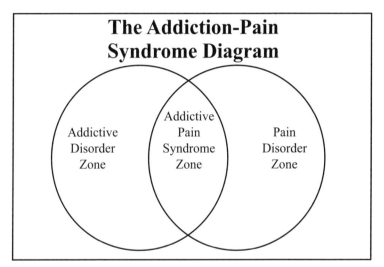

The Addiction-Pain Syndrome Diagram

Addictive Disorder Zone

Addictive Pain Syndrome Zone

Pain Disorder Zone

There are seven basic recovery activities described below that will address these zones. They are essential habits of good, healthy living. Anyone who wants to live a responsible, healthy, and fulfilling life will get in the habit of regularly doing these things.

For people in recovery, these activities are essential. For those who also have a chronic pain disorder (Addiction Pain Syndrome), these steps become even more crucial. A regular schedule of these activities—designed to match patients' unique profiles of recovery needs, pain management requirements, and high-risk situations—is necessary for their brains and bodies to heal from the damage caused by addiction and the chronic pain condition.

Patients are instructed to read the following list of recovery activities and identify which activities they think will be helpful for their recovery and pain management program. They are asked to notice the obstacles they face in doing them on a regular basis and indicate their strategies to overcome those obstacles. They are then asked if they are willing to put the activities on their recovery plan.

The seven recovery activities are listed in the following table.

Exercise Eight, Part 1:
Selecting Your Recovery Activities

Having a plan for each day will help your recovery and enable you to practice better pain management. People who successfully recover and effectively manage their pain tend to do certain things. These recovery principles are proven. In A.A. there is such a strong belief in them that many people with solid recovery will say, "If you want what we have, do what we did!" and "It works if you work it!" The same applies to pain management; those who are most effective with pain management have learned to develop a recovery/management plan. However, not everyone does exactly the same things. Once you understand yourself and the basic principles of recovery, pain management, and relapse prevention, you can build an effective personalized program for yourself.

When people first read the following list, they tend to get defensive. "I can't do all of those things!" they say to themselves. I invite you to think about your recovery as if you were hiking in the Grand Canyon and had to jump across a ravine that was about three feet wide and 100 feet deep. It's better to jump three feet too far than to risk jumping one inch too short. The same is true of recovery. It's better to plan to do a little bit more than you need to do than to risk not doing enough. In A.A. they say, "Half measures availed us nothing!"

The seven basic recovery activities described below are actually habits of good, healthy living. Anyone who wants to live a responsible, healthy, and fulfilling life will get in the habit of regularly doing these things. For people in recovery these activities are essential, and if you also have a chronic pain condition, these steps become even more crucial. A regular schedule of these activities, designed to match your unique profile of recovery needs, pain management requirements, and high-risk situations, is necessary for your brain and body to heal from the damage by medication use and your chronic pain condition.

Instructions:
Read the following list of recovery activities and identify which activities you think will be helpful for your recovery and pain management program. Notice the obstacles you face in doing them on a regular basis, and indicate your strategies to overcome those obstacles.

1. **Professional Counseling:** The success of your recovery and effective pain management will depend on regular attendance at education sessions, group therapy sessions, and/or individual therapy or counseling sessions. The scientific literature on treatment effectiveness clearly shows that the more you invest in professional counseling and/or therapy during the first two years of recovery, the more likely you are to stay in recovery. This process needs to include pain management treatment planning.

    A. Do I believe that I need to do this?
        ❐ Yes ❐ No ❐ Unsure   Please explain:
    B. The obstacles that might prevent me from doing this are:
    C. Possible ways of overcoming these obstacles are:
    D. Will I put this on my recovery plan?
        ❐ Yes ❐ No ❐ Unsure   Please explain:

2. **Self-Help Programs:** There are a number of self-help programs—such as Alcoholics Anonymous (A.A.), Pills Anonymous (P.A.), Chronic Pain Anonymous (C.P.A.), Chronic Pain Support Groups, Narcotics Anonymous (N.A.), Rational Recovery, and Women for Sobriety—that can support you in your efforts to live a sober and responsible life. These programs all have several things in common: (1) They ask you to abstain from inappropriate mood-altering substances and to live a responsible life; (2) they encourage you to regularly attend meetings, so you can meet and develop relationships with other people living sober and responsible lives; (3) they ask you to attend regularly with an established member of the group (usually called a sponsor) who will help you learn about the organization and get through the rough spots; and (4) they promote a program of recovery (often in the form of steps or structured exercises for you to work on outside of meetings) that focuses on techniques for changing your thinking, emotional management, urge management, and behavior.

Scientific research shows that the more committed and actively involved you are in self-help groups during the first two years of recovery, the greater your ability to avoid relapse. You should also consider joining a chronic pain support group, because research indicated personal empowerment is crucial for developing effective, long-term chronic pain management.

A. Do I believe that I need to do this?
  ❏ Yes ❏ No ❏ Unsure   Please explain:

B. The obstacles that might prevent me from this are:

C. Possible ways of overcoming these obstacles are:

D. Will I put this on my recovery plan?
  ❏ Yes ❏ No ❏ Unsure   Please explain:

3. **Proper Diet:** What you eat can affect how you think, feel, and act. Many chemically dependent people find they feel better if they eat three well-balanced meals a day, use vitamin and amino-acid supplements, avoid eating sugar and foods made with white flour, and cut back on or stop smoking cigarettes and drinking beverages containing caffeine, such as coffee and colas. Recovering people who do not follow these simple principles of healthy diet and meal planning tend to feel anxious and depressed, have strong and violent mood swings, feel constantly angry and resentful, and periodically experience powerful cravings. They're more likely to relapse. Those who follow a proper diet tend to feel better and have lower relapse rates. Proper nutrition is also crucial for effective pain management.

A. Do I believe that I need to do this?
  ❏ Yes ❏ No ❏ Unsure   Please explain:

B. The obstacles that might prevent me from doing this are:

C. Possible ways of overcoming these obstacles are:

D. Will I put this on my recovery plan?
  ❏ Yes ❏ No ❏ Unsure   Please explain:

4. **Exercise Program:** If your chronic pain permits, doing thirty minutes of aerobic exercise each day will help your brain recover and help you feel better about yourself. Fast walking, jogging, swimming, and aerobic classes are all beneficial. It's also helpful to do strength-building exercises (such as weight lifting) and flexibility exercises (such as stretching) in addition to the aerobic exercise. You need to work with your doctor or health-care practitioner to determine the most effective (and safest)

exercise program for you. Many pain management providers state that flexibility and mobility are essential for effective pain management.

A. Do I believe that I need to do this?

❏ Yes ❏ No ❏ Unsure Please explain:

B. The obstacles that might prevent me from doing this are:

C. Possible ways of overcoming these obstacles are:

D. Will I put this on my recovery plan?

❏ Yes ❏ No ❏ Unsure Please explain:

5. **Stress Management Program:** Stress is a major cause of relapse. In addition, as you read earlier in this book, an increase in stress often leads to an increase in pain. Recovering people who learn how to manage stress without using self-defeating behaviors tend to stay in recovery and learn how to more effectively manage their chronic pain symptoms. Those who do not learn to manage stress tend to relapse or suffer more with their pain. Stress management involves learning relaxation exercises and taking quiet time on a daily basis to relax. It also involves long hours of working and taking time for recreation and relaxation. Meditation can also be part of this program.

A. Do I believe that I need to do this?

❏ Yes ❏ No ❏ Unsure Please explain:

B. The obstacles that might prevent me from doing this are:

C. Possible ways of overcoming these obstacles are:

D. Will I put this on my recovery plan?

❏ Yes ❏ No ❏ Unsure Please explain:

6. **Spiritual Development Program:** Human beings have both a physical self (based on the health of our brains and bodies) and a nonphysical self (based on the health of our value systems and spiritual lives). Most recovering people find they need to invest regular time in developing themselves spiritually (in other words, exercising the nonphysical aspects of who they are). Twelve-Step programs, like A.A., provide an excellent program for spiritual recovery, as do many communities of faith and spiritual programs. At the heart of any spiritual program are three activities: (1) fellowship, where you spend time talking with other people who use similar methods; (2) private prayer and meditation, where you take time to be conscious of yourself in the presence of your Higher Power or to consciously reflect

on your spiritual self; and (3) group worship, where you pray and meditate with other people who share a similar spiritual philosophy.

A. Do I believe that I need to do this?
   ☐ Yes ☐ No ☐ Unsure Please explain:

B. The obstacles that might prevent me from doing this are:

C. Possible ways of overcoming these obstacles are:

D. Will I put this on my recovery plan?
   ☐ Yes ☐ No ☐ Unsure Please explain:

7. **Morning and Evening Inventories:** People who avoid relapse and successfully obtain lifelong recovery learn how to break free of automatic and unconscious self-defeating responses. They learn to live consciously each day, being aware of what they're doing and taking responsibility for what they do and its consequences. To stay consciously aware, they take time each morning to plan their day (a morning planning inventory) and they take time each evening to review their progress and problems (an evening review inventory). They discuss what they learn about themselves with other people who are involved in their recovery program.

For people with chronic pain, it is important to keep a pain journal that identifies stress and trigger patterns as well as associated thoughts, feelings, and behaviors. During times of increased pain, keeping a daily pain journal is essential, leading to more effective pain management. Incorporating the Identifying and Rating the Severity of Your Pain Symptoms worksheet from Exercise One in this book would be an important addition to your pain journaling.

A. Do I believe that I need to do this?
   ☐ Yes ☐ No ☐ Unsure Please explain:

B. The obstacles that might prevent me from doing this are:

C. Possible ways of overcoming these obstacles are:

D. Will I put this on my recovery plan?
   ☐ Yes ☐ No ☐ Unsure Please explain:

Exercise Eight, Part 2:
Completing Your Schedule of Recovery Activities

Once patients have identified the recovery activities they will use to avoid relapse, they develop a schedule of those activities. Part 2 of Exercise Eight assists patients by introducing a weekly planner. A reproduction of this exercise is in the following table.

Instructions

On the next page is a weekly planner (see workbook, p. 84) that will allow you to create a schedule of weekly recovery and pain management activities. Think of a typical week and enter the pain management and recovery activities that you plan to routinely schedule in the correct time slot for each day. Recovery activities and/or pain management activities are specific things that you do at scheduled times on certain days. If you can't enter the activity on a daily planner at a specific time, it's not a recovery and/or pain management activity. Most people find it helpful to have more than one scheduled activity for each day.

Remember, recovery activities fall into four quadrants:

- **Biological:** This quadrant includes activities that improve the health of your physical self. Some examples include abstinence from inappropriate medications, regularly scheduled balanced meals, scheduled exercise regimen, physical therapy appointments, daily hygiene, etc.

- **Psychological:** This quadrant includes activities that help you identify and change negative thinking patterns and cope with uncomfortable emotions. Some examples include counseling/therapy appointments, reading recovery literature, anger management training, etc.

- **Social:** This quadrant includes activities that help you let go of enabling or addiction-prone relationships and encourages developing relationships with recovery-prone people who will support your recovery. Some examples include finding an appropriate sponsor who understands both the pain management and chemical recovery processes; and saying goodbye to problem people, places, and things that could trigger relapse, etc.

- **Spiritual:** This quadrant includes activities that will help you develop or improve your relationship with your inner self or Higher Power. Some examples include prayer and meditation, visits to nature, attending religious or spiritual services, etc.

The examples above are only a starting place. You need to develop your own personalized recovery schedule. It needs to contain activities that will help you identify and manage problem high-risk situations without putting you at risk of using inappropriate pain medication, including alcohol or other drugs, or cutting back or eliminating effective pain management activities.

Once patients have developed the calendar, Part 3 of Exercise Eight is used to test the scheduled events. Patients are asked to complete the exercise listed in the following table.

Exercise Eight, Part 3:
Testing Your Schedule of Recovery Activities

Instructions

1. Go back and review the primary high-risk situation that you want your recovery and pain management program to help you identify and manage. Read the personal title and description and the thought, feeling, urge, and action statements carefully. What is the personal title and description of this high-risk situation?

Title: _____

Description: *I know that I'm in a high-risk situation when I ...*

2. Review your Weekly Planner. What is the most important recovery and/or pain management activity that will help you manage your high-risk situation?

   A. How can you use your recovery and/or pain management activity to help you identify your high-risk situation should it occur? (Remember, most high-risk situations develop in an automatic and unconscious way. A trigger is activated, and you start using the old ways of thinking and acting without being consciously aware of what you are doing. To prevent relapse it's helpful to regularly schedule recovery and/or pain management activities that will encourage you to talk about how you are thinking, feeling, and acting, and then receive feedback if you experience high-risk situations.)

B. If you start to experience your high-risk situation again, how can you use this recovery activity to manage it? (Remember, managing a high-risk situation means changing how you think, feel, and act. How can this recovery activity help you stop thinking and doing things that make you feel like relapsing? How can it help you start thinking and doing things that make you want to get back into recovery?)

3. Review your Weekly Planner again. What is the second most important recovery activity that will help you manage your high-risk situation?

A. How can you use this recovery activity to help you identify your high-risk situation should it occur?

B. If you start to experience your high-risk situation again, how can you use this recovery activity to manage it?

4. Review your Weekly Planner one last time. What is the third most important recovery activity that will help you manage your high-risk situation?

A. How can you use this recovery activity to help you identify your high-risk situation should it occur?

B. If you start to experience your high-risk situation again, how can you use this recovery activity to manage it?

5. What other recovery activities can you think of that could be more effective in helping you identify and manage future high-risk situations should they occur?

The next chapter covers the measurement of treatment outcomes as well as discussing the last exercise in the *Addiction-Free Pain Management™ Workbook*, which is a final evaluation for the patient. While Exercise Nine is not a clinical process, per se, it is an important indicator of treatment success or problems. It also allows patients to experience a profound sense of accomplishment.

By the time Jean and Dean reached the end of the workbook exercises they were both fairly stable. Dean did experience a brief and minor relapse episode related to a very emotional couple's therapy session where he finally talked about his affairs. Fortunately, he immediately used his relapse intervention plan with his relapse prevention network to quickly restabilize.

Jean did not relapse, but her life became very stressful and she needed to backtrack into some basic self-care treatment planning. In addition, both patients were encouraged to start working in the *Denial Management Counseling for Effective Pain Management* workbook and then move on to the *Relapse Prevention Therapy Workbook* as soon as they were stable. Their progress in those processes will be covered in future publications.

> An ounce of relapse prevention planning
> is worth a pound of treatment cure.

The important thing to remember with relapse prevention is the old saying, "An ounce of prevention is worth a pound of cure." Patients must be educated to get and stay active with their recovery and not wait until after they are in a relapse mode.

It is helpful to have patients look at a relapse prevention plan like a car insurance policy. Many people are fortunate not to collect on that insurance, but it sure is nice to know that it will be available when they need it. A solid relapse prevention plan works the same way. A patient may never need to use the interventions they set up, but should they start that downward spiral, it is comforting for them to know they have a plan in place that will support them and put the brakes on relapse.

> Relapse prevention is simple but not easy.

Like many other things in recovery, relapse prevention is simple—*but not easy*. And although relapse prevention is an inside job, that does not mean patients have to do it alone. Help is out there for those who need it, want it, and reach out for it.

However, chronic pain patients have a much better chance of quality recovery when their healthcare providers use a combination of the APM™ *Core Clinical Exercises*, combined with as-needed *Medication Management Components*, and implementing appropriate *Nonpharmacological Treatment Processes*. It is the healthcare providers' responsibility to be aware of all potential resources in their communities.

In the next chapter you will learn Jean and Dean's self-evaluation outcomes, which is the final exercise in the *Addiction-Free Pain Management™ Workbook*. This exercise is also described in the final chapter and is designed to help patients complete a final evaluation to learn how much they have benefited from all their work. This is also a useful tool for clinicians to determine the effectiveness of the treatment process.

- **Call to Action for the Ninth Chapter**

It is time to summarize what you learned so far now that you have come to the end of the ninth chapter. Please answer the questions below.

1. What is the most important thing you learned about yourself and your ability to help addicted pain patients as a result of completing Chapter Nine?

2. What are you willing to commit to do differently as a result of what you have learned by completing this chapter?

3. What obstacles might get in the way of making these changes? What can you do to overcome these roadblocks?

**Take time to pause and reflect, then
go to the next page to review Chapter Ten.**

Chapter Ten
Measuring Treatment Effectiveness

Determining the effectiveness of chemical dependency treatment is relatively straightforward. If the patient remains abstinent from alcohol and other psychoactive drugs, the treatment is deemed successful. Determining the outcome of chronic pain treatment is much more complex.

It is not enough for chemically dependent chronic pain patients to achieve abstinence; they must also experience an improvement in their pain condition and quality of life. In addition, they must have a solid relapse prevention and pain management plan in place that continues to be evaluated and modified frequently.

- **Benchmarks for Effective Treatment**

Follow-up data should be gathered at different intervals, using specific benchmarks that gauge successful treatment outcomes. The first follow-up occurs at the completion of primary treatment, followed by testing at three months, six months, nine months, and one year.

These benchmarks include assessing improvement in quality of life. Improvements are determined by such factors as the patient returning to work or other significant increases in the quality of life, as well as the absence or significant reduction of psychoactive drug use. Family members and significant others must be contacted for their input. Blood testing should be performed to verify the addictive medication report.

To be considered a total treatment success the following criteria must be met: After one year a patient must not be taking any inappropriate chemicals, report an increase in their quality of life, and report a decrease both in their inactivity due to pain and in their pain levels. However, it is important to realize that in some cases the most optimal outcome will be a reduction in the problematic medication, not total elimination.

Successful APM™ Treatment Criteria

- Reduction or elimination of inappropriate medication
- Pain symptoms are decreased
- Inactivity due to pain is decreased
- Quality of life is increased

Utilizing the Pain Outcome Profile (POP) Instrument

A relatively new instrument, the *Pain Outcome Profile* (POP), was developed by the American Academy of Pain Management and Drs. Michael Clark and Ron Gironda at the James A. Haley Veterans Hospital in Tampa, Florida.

The POP assesses three domains of a patient's pain experience with twenty core clinical items: pain perception, perceived physical impairment due to pain, and several aspects of emotional functioning. These domains are assessed using two pain intensity scales, three self-reports of functional impairment scales, and two scales that address self-reported emotional functioning (seven scales total).

According to information on the American Academy of Pain Management (AAPM) Web site (*http://www.aapainmanage.org*), the use of the Pain Outcome Profile will assist programs in preparing to comply with standards put in place by the Joint Commission on Accreditation of Healthcare Organizations (JCAHO) in 2001. These standards require healthcare providers to

- recognize the right of patients to receive appropriate assessment and management of pain;
- establish the existence of pain and assess its nature and intensity in all patients;
- record the results of the assessment in a way that facilitates regular reassessment and follow-up;
- determine and assure staff competency in pain assessment and management and address pain assessment and management in the orientation of all new staff;
- establish policies and procedures that support the appropriate prescription or ordering of effective pain medications;
- educate patients and their families about effective pain management; and

- address patient needs for symptom management in the discharge planning process.

Finally, according to the AAPM, the POP can assist programs in meeting standards established by the Commission on Accreditation of Rehabilitation Facilities (CARF) for Information and Outcomes Management Systems.

Measuring outcomes allows for the enhancement of clinical services through a process of continuous quality improvement. Patients and third-party payers alike increasingly demand accountability on the part of treatment providers, and use of the POP may be one component of your program's overall outcomes measurement strategy.

• Evaluating Pain and Addiction Management Skills

Patients also need to be given an effective method to evaluate and rate their own progress for overall pain and addiction recovery. On page 88 in the *Addiction-Free Pain Management™ Workbook* you will find such a tool. After completing the first eight clinical exercises in the workbook, patients then have a chance to complete a final evaluation. The following table gives the process they are instructed to complete.

Completing Your Final Evaluation Exercise

Instructions

The ultimate test of whether you have benefited from completing the exercises in this workbook will be your ability to increase effective pain management and avoid relapse. It may be helpful, however, to review what you have accomplished. A careful evaluation may help you identify areas in your Relapse Prevention Plan that are incomplete. By going back and completing these areas, you may avoid unnecessary relapse and the resulting pain and problems.

Here is a checklist that can help you decide if you have accomplished the objectives of completing this workbook. Read each statement and ask yourself if you have fully completed that objective, partially completed it, or not completed it at all. Remember, this is a self-evaluation designed to help you determine if you have the skills needed to avoid relapse. Be honest with yourself. If you relapse because you haven't learned

---

the skills to stay in recovery, you are the one who will pay the price.

1. ***Understanding Your Pain:*** I understand and can explain the common effects of my chronic pain, the main effects that I personally experienced, and can differentiate between my pysical and psychological/emotional pain symptoms.

   Level of Completion:
   ❐ None (0)   ❐ Partial (5)   ❐ Full (10)   Score (0–10) ___

2. ***The Effects of Prescription and/or Other Drugs (Including Alcohol):*** I understand and can explain the benefits I obtained from using prescription or other drugs, and what I wanted to get from using these chemicals. I can also understand and explain the problems I experienced as a result of using.

   Level of Completion:
   ❐ None (0)   ❐ Partial (5)   ❐ Full (10)   Score (0–10) ___

3. ***Decision Making about Pain Medication:*** I understand and can explain the reasons I started using pain medication, alcohol, or other drugs inappropriately. I understand and can explain the reasons why I stopped using pain medication, including alcohol and other drugs, as well as what I did to adhere to my medication agreement.

   Level of Completion:
   ❐ None (0)   ❐ Partial (5)   ❐ Full (10)   Score (0–10) ___

4. ***Moving into the Solution:*** I can define what my medication management agreement and recovery plan includes. I have completed and signed a medication management agreement, committing to maintain adherence to the plan and practice effective pain management. I have developed a relapse prevention intervention plan that describes the responsibilities for me, my counselor, and significant others (two or three) to stop relapse quickly should it occur.

   Level of Completion:
   ❐ None (0)   ❐ Partial (5)   ❐ Full (10)   Score (0–10) ___

5. ***Identifying High-Risk Situations:*** I am able to identify the immediate high-risk situations that can cause me to use inappropriate pain medication (including alcohol) or other drugs and/or stop using an effective pain management program despite my commitment not to by developing an Initial High-Risk Situation List and identifying my immediate high-risk situations.

Level of Completion:
☐ None (0) ☐ Partial (5) ☐ Full (10) Score (0–10) ___

6. ***Personalizing High-Risk Situations:*** I am able to concretely and specifically describe the immediate high-risk situations, having developed meaningful personal titles and personal descriptions.

Level of Completion:
☐ None (0) ☐ Partial (5) ☐ Full (10) Score (0–10) ___

7. ***Mapping Past Mismanaged High-Risk Situations:*** I am able to use Situation Mapping to objectively describe past high-risk situations that were managed in a way that led to using inappropriate pain medication (including alcohol) or other drugs and/or ineffective pain management.

Level of Completion:
☐ None (0) ☐ Partial (5) ☐ Full (10) Score (0–10) ___

8. ***Analyzing Past Mismanaged High-Risk Situations:*** I am able to use High-Risk Situation Analysis to identify the thoughts, feelings, urges, actions, and relationship patterns caused by the past mismanagement of the high-risk situation.

Level of Completion:
☐ None (0) ☐ Partial (5) ☐ Full (10) Score (0–10) ___

9. ***Managing High-Risk Thoughts and Feelings:*** I am able to (1) identify the general way of thinking that is driving situation management; (2) show the relationship between these thoughts and the feelings driving this mismanagement; and (3) use positive self-talk techniques to challenge the thoughts and feelings driving situation mismanagement.

Level of Completion:
☐ None (0) ☐ Partial (5) ☐ Full (10) Score (0–10) ___

10. ***Developing a Recovery Plan:*** I am able to develop a schedule of recovery activities that will support my ongoing identification and management of high-risk situations and help me to intervene early should I be tempted to violate my medication management agreement and/or use ineffective pain management.

Level of Completion:
☐ None (0) ☐ Partial (5) ☐ Full (10) Score (0–10) ___

11. ***Overall Skill Level:*** I have developed an overall ability to identify and manage my high-risk situations that lead me from sta-

bility to violating my medication management agreement and/ or ineffective pain management. I have developed a schedule of recovery activities that will support my ongoing high-risk situation identification and management.

Level of Completion:
❏ None (0) ❏ Partial (5) ❏ Full (10)   Score (0–10) ___

Although the above exercise can be an effective benchmark for patients to evaluate themselves, follow-up sessions are needed to determine the ongoing effectiveness of treatment.

• **A New Beginning**

Using the APM™ System increases positive treatment outcomes.

The Road Map to APM™ Recovery

APM™ recovery utilizes detailed, accurate assessments followed by multidimensional treatment plans. These treatment plans include the *Core Clinical Exercises* and, when needed, the *Medication Management Components*. They also include the *Nonpharmacological Treatment Processes,* as well as the proven CENAPS® relapse prevention protocols. These methods are implemented to help ensure ongoing recovery.

An Integrated APM™ Treatment Approach
* Core clinical exercises
* Medication management components
* Nonpharmacological treatment processes

More and more patients are benefiting from the implementation of APM™ methodologies than from either traditional chemical dependency treatment or pain management care at chronic pain clinics. These patients are able to resume healthy and productive lives and experience an overall improved quality of life.

This was the case for Jean; she stopped using all of her problematic pain medication and her family relationships improved. In addition, she continued to build trust and safety in her women's group and is working an effective pain management program.

Dean, however, continues to struggle but has learned some valuable lessons from his recent relapse. He is much more hopeful, now, that he will eventually succeed in becoming a high-functioning member of society. His prognosis has significantly improved as a result of the APM™ process. Based on his current signs of progress, he should become totally stabilized and move into a healthy, ongoing recovery.

Spreading the Word—APM™ Works

As you take your patients through the APM™ system, you become part of the solution that offers understanding, hope, and recovery to an underserved population that still suffers. This is a new beginning. My challenge to you is to take what you have learned, integrate it, network with other treatment professionals, and share it—*APM™ works!*

- **The Final Call to Action for Managing Pain and Coexisting Disorders**

It is time to summarize what you learned now that you have come to the end of the final chapter. Please answer the questions below.

1. What is the most important thing you learned about yourself and your ability to help addicted pain patients as a result of completing this book?

2. What are you willing to commit to do differently as a result of what you have learned by completing this book?

3. What obstacles might get in the way of making these changes? What can you do to overcome these roadblocks?

You have now finished *Managing Pain and Coexisting Disorders* and the core components of the Addiction-Free Pain Management system. Go to the next page to review information in the Appendix.

Appendix

- **The APM™ Strategic Treatment Plan**

A. **Problem Title:** High Risk of Ineffective Pain Management and/or Inappropriate Medication Use

B. **Problem Description:** The client has made a commitment to abstain from problematic pain medication (including alcohol) and other drugs for a period of time and is facing a number of immediate high-risk situations that could cause inappropriate medication use and/or ineffective pain management despite that commitment.

C. **Goal:** The client will be able to adhere to their *medication management agreement* and continue with effective pain management by identifying and effectively managing the immediate high-risk situations that can cause relapse.

   Start Date: ____   *Target Date:* ____   *Actual Date:* ____

D. **Interventions:** The client will participate in a combination of group and individual therapy sessions, psychoeducation sessions, supervised study halls, and self-help group meetings where the following interventions will be implemented:

(1) **The APM™ Treatment Contract:** The client will complete an evaluation of presenting problems, meet the admission criteria for Addiction-Free Pain Management™ (APM™), review the basic APM™ procedures, and agree to the *APM™ Treatment Contract*.

   Start Date: ____   *Target Date:* ____   *Actual Date:* ____

   Resources: _____

   _____

   Assisted By: _____

   _____

Level of Completion:
❏ Full ❏ Partial ❏ None *Completion Score (0–10):* ___
Notes: _____

_____

(2) **The Medication Management Agreement:** The client will agree to abstain from problematic pain medication (including alcohol) and other drugs for the duration of treatment to complete alcohol and drug testing on a random basis or if requested for any reason by their healthcare provider(s).

Start Date: _____   *Target Date:* _____   *Actual Date:* _____

Resources: _____

_____

Assisted By: _____

_____

Level of Completion:
❏ Full ❏ Partial ❏ None   *Completion Score (0–10):* ___

Notes: _____

_____

(3) **Relapse Early Intervention Plan:** The client will complete a relapse early intervention plan that describes the responsibilities of the client, counselor, and significant others to stop relapse quickly should it occur. The client will also develop a craving intervention plan and a pain flare-up plan.

Start Date: _____   *Target Date:* _____   *Actual Date:* _____

Resources: _____

_____

Assisted By: _____

_____

Level of Completion:
❏ Full ❏ Partial ❏ None   *Completion Score (0–10):* ___

Notes: _____

_____

(4) **Identifying and Personalizing High-Risk Situations:** The client will identify immediate high-risk situations that can cause the use of problematic pain medication (including alcohol) and other drugs despite their commitment not to. They will review the high-risk situation list and write a personal title and descriptions for use in self-monitoring.

Start Date: ____   *Target Date:* ____   *Actual Date:* ____

Resources: _____

_____

Assisted By: _____

_____

Level of Completion:
☐ Full   ☐ Partial   ☐ None   *Completion Score (0–10):* ___

Notes: _____

_____

(5) **Mapping High-Risk Situations:** The client will objectively describe past and future high-risk situations that were mismanaged in a way that led to use of problematic pain medication (including alcohol) and other drugs and identify new and more effective management strategies.

Start Date: ____   *Target Date:* ____   *Actual Date:* ____

Resources: _____

_____

Assisted By: _____

_____

Level of Completion:
☐ Full   ☐ Partial   ☐ None   *Completion Score (0–10):* ___

Notes: _____

_____

(6) **Analyzing and Managing High-Risk Situations:** The client will identify the thoughts, feelings, urges, actions, and reactions of others (TFUARs) related to managing each high-risk situation in a way that leads to using problematic pain medication (including alcohol) and other drugs and identify new and more effective TFUARs.

Start Date: ____   *Target Date:* ____   *Actual Date:* ____

Resources: _____

_____

Assisted By: _____

Level of Completion:
❏ Full ❏ Partial ❏ None *Completion Score (0–10):* ___
Notes: _____

_____

(7) **Recovery Planning:** The client will develop a schedule of recovery activities that supports the ongoing identification and
sober/responsible management of future high-risk situations.

   Start Date: ___   *Target Date:* ___   *Actual Date:* ___

   Resources: _____

   _____

   Assisted By: _____

   _____

Level of Completion:
❏ Full ❏ Partial ❏ None *Completion Score (0–10):* ___
Notes: _____

_____

(8) **Overall Response:** The client has developed the overall ability to anticipate, identify, and responsibly manage critical
high-risk situations without using problematic pain medication (including alcohol) and other drugs and/or adhering to
their effective pain management program.

   Notes: _____

   _____

   _____

   _____

Overall Level of Completion:
❏ Full ❏ Partial ❏ None *Completion Score (0–10):* ___

• Red Flags for Pain Medication Addiction

By Dr. Stephen F. Grinstead, LMFT, ACRPS

Differentiating between appropriate use of pain medication and the beginning of abuse can sometimes be difficult for healthcare providers or their patients to determine. There are progressive stages of problematic use including medication dependency, medication abuse, pseudoaddiction, and finally addiction. The confusion and uncertainty of this progression is a challenge for both the patient and the treatment provider.

Many people in chronic pain are afraid to take their narcotic medication, because they have heard horror stories of people getting hooked on pain pills. This leads to their choosing to be undermedicated and they end up suffering. If the person happens to be in recovery for alcoholism or another drug addiction, the problem is even worse. If these people undermedicate, it could trigger a relapse. Of course the other side of the coin is if they are overmedicated, it could also lead to rapid tolerance building and finally reactivation of their addiction.

Following is a list of *red flags* or indicators that someone is using their pain medication in a manner that could eventually lead to problems or even addiction. Both treatment providers and their patients need to be familiar with these red flags and to seek professional help from a person trained in addiction who also has experience, understanding, or training in pain management.

Instructions: *Review each of the items below and rate each on a 0 to 10 scale with 0 meaning this item is not and has not been a problem to 10 meaning this is a serious problem.*

☐ 1. After adjusting to the medication the patient still experiences a sense of euphoria.

☐ 2. The patient seems to have a preoccupation with their pain medication.

☐ 3. The patient has urges or cravings about their pain medication.

☐ 4. There is an abnormal increase in tolerance requiring frequent increases in dose.

☐ 5. There is a decrease in the patient's nonpharmacological pain management activities.

☐ 6. The patient is using nonprescribed substances including alcohol and/or other drugs: marijuana, over-the-counter analgesics, methamphetamine, etc.

☐ 7. The patient is unable to take their pain medication as prescribed—type, quantity, and/or frequency.

☐ 8. The patient is experiencing problems with cognition, affect, and/or behavior.

☐ 9. The patient's quality of life and/or relationships are being negatively impacted by their use of pain medication.

☐ 10. The patient continues problematic use of medication despite negative consequences.

☐ 11. The patient uses medications in physically dangerous situations: driving a car, operating power tools, providing child care to young children, etc.

☐ 12. The client experiences withdrawal symptoms if they go too long between doses or stop their medication abruptly.

☐ 13. The patient is experiencing medication-related legal problems.

☐ 14. The patient is not informing one healthcare provider what medication another provider is prescribing.

☐ 15. The patient has a history—or family history—of alcoholism or other drug addiction.

☐ 16. The patient is using the medication to cope with psychological/emotional type pain or to cope with stressful or uncomfortable situations.

☐ 17. Family members or friends report concerns about the patient's use of medication.

☐ 18. The patient self-reports that they believe they are having problems with their medication.

☐ 19. The patient is unable to fulfill major obligations with family, friends, and/or work due to their use of medication.

☐ 20. The patient frequently needs early refills and may rationalize this by coming up with sometimes unusual excuses: I lost it, someone else took it, it fell in the water, etc.

☐ 21. The patient is resistant to referrals for psychological assessment and/or treatment.

☐ 22. The patient is resistant to nonnarcotic medications or referrals for nonmedication type pain management interventions or makes excuses why they won't work.

☐ 23. The patient is resistant to sign consent to release forms allowing their provider to discuss their treatment with other healthcare providers they have been seeing.

Some of the items above may be difficult to determine, which is why collaboration is so essential. This collaboration should include the patient, the patient's support network, other healthcare providers, or any other sources that could help gain the needed information. If several of the red-flag areas have scores above a 5, or a few have scores in the 8–10 range, it is time for a referral to an appropriate addiction specialist to make a more accurate assessment of a potential medication abuse/addiction problem. You can also follow up by using the Medication Problem Checklist from the *Addiction-Free Pain Management™ Workbook.*

• A Guide for Managing Pain Medication in Recovery

Developed By: Dr. Stephen F. Grinstead, LMFT, ACRPS, and Sheila Thares, RN, MSN, APNP

For someone in recovery for chemical dependency the use of mood-altering prescription medication can and does lead to relapse. The primary goal of this worksheet is for you to learn how to develop a plan that will prevent sabotaging an effective recovery program, while at the same time learning to avoid other addiction problems or a destructive pattern of relapse. Relapse includes ineffective pain management and/or abuse of your pain medication.

This worksheet is a result of many years of study, researching literature on outcome-based treatment, and personal experience. It is designed for people recovering from any chemical dependency who are facing an invasive surgical procedure (medical or dental) that could entail the use of psychoactive medication. It is also intended for others who may not be in recovery, but have some risk factors for dependency and want to avoid becoming chemically dependent. Included in this publication are some strategic action steps you can take to safely and effectively prepare yourself for an upcoming surgical procedure.

To accomplish these goals you will need to do more than just read this worksheet. You will need to discuss your responses to each of the following guidelines with someone who can help you sort out the thoughts and feelings that may come as a result of these exercises. If you don't have a counselor, you can do this work with the assistance of a self-help group sponsor who is willing to support you through this process. **Discussing what you're learning from this process with another person or a group of people will improve your ability to develop a plan that will prevent relapse.**

When a person is in recovery for chemical dependency, whether the substance be prescription drugs, alcohol, marijuana, etc., the risk of relapse is always present. One issue that tends to be especially problematic and a relapse trigger for recovering alcoholics and/or addicts is pain. It is unrealistic to expect that we will never have a medical or dental situation where pain management is needed. In addition, if the person in recovery also suffers from a chronic pain condition, relapse prevention becomes even more crucial. Here are some guidelines for people in recovery who want to minimize their risk of relapse.

263

1. During early recovery postpone nonurgent dental work (except prevention or restorative) and elective surgical procedures requiring mind-altering medications. When you do need to be on medication, make sure that an addiction medicine practitioner/specialist is used for consultation and/or prescribing that medication.

2. If you need to be on medication, have your sponsor, significant other, or an appropriate support person hold and dispense the medication. Keep only a twenty-four-hour supply available.

3. Consult with an addiction medicine practitioner/specialist about using nonaddictive medications such as anti-inflammatory, or other over-the-counter analgesics.

4. Be open to exploring all nonchemical pain management modalities. Some of the more common ones are acupuncture, chiropractic, physical therapy, massage therapy, and hydrotherapy. In addition, identifying and managing uncomfortable emotions may also decrease your pain significantly.

5. Be aware of your stress levels, and have a stress management program in place such as meditation, exercise, relaxation, music, etc. If you lower your stress, you will usually lower your pain as a result.

6. Take personal responsibility to augment your support group meetings in order to decrease isolation, as well as urges and cravings.

7. Inform all of your healthcare providers about being in recovery, and be aware of the importance of consulting with an addiction medicine practitioner/specialist in the event mind-altering medication is needed. There may be times you need to be on medication, but the risk of relapse can be minimized if open communication is maintained between the addiction medicine practitioner/specialist, yourself, and other healthcare providers.

8. Do not overwork, especially if you are in pain or sick. Add one extra day off to your return-to-work plan to avoid fatigue and promote healing.

9. Be open and aware of the cross-addiction concept. Decline helpful offers to use someone else's prescriptions. Any psychoactive chemical could trigger a relapse of your addiction because all mood-altering drugs enter the limbic system as dopamine. This explains why nonpolyaddicted alcoholics can relapse to alcohol after receiving opiates.

10. Because depression is common for people with chronic pain, be open to the possibility of taking appropriate antidepressants if needed.

11. Be aware of the importance of proper nutrition and exercise as an important part of chronic pain recovery. Stretch slowly at first, then structure progressive walking at least once a day, or twice if necessary, to complete the designated distance. Increase the distance as you are able. Add strengthening exercises if cleared by your healthcare provider. Remember, protein assists repair of injuries; therefore, it is important to create a nutrition plan for tissue repair.

12. Explore your past beliefs and role models from childhood regarding pain and pain management. Look for healthy role models for pain management in recovery.

- *Pain Management Reference List and Recommended Reading List*

Barrett, S., et al. (2006). *Consumer health: A guide to intelligent decisions.* Columbus, OH: McGraw-Hill.

Boriskin, J. (2004). *PTSD and addiction: A practical guide for clinicians and counselors.* Center City, MN: Hazelden.

Carr, D., Loeser, J., & Morris, D. (2005). *Narrative, pain, and suffering.* Seattle, WA: IASP Press.

Catalano, E., & Hardin, K. (1996). *The chronic pain control workbook: A step-by-step guide for coping with and overcoming pain.* Oakland, CA: New Harbinger.

Caudill, M. (2001). *Managing pain before it manages you.* New York: Guilford Press.

Cleveland, M. (1999). *Chronic illness and the twelve steps: A practical approach to spiritual resilience.* Center City, MN: Hazelden.

Colvin, R. (2002). *Prescription drug addiction: The hidden epidemic.* Omaha, NE: Addicus Books.

Corey, D., & Solomon, S. (1989). *Pain: Free yourself for life.* New York: Penguin Books USA.

Davis, M., Eshelman, E.R., & McKay, M. (1995). *The relaxation and stress reduction workbook, fourth edition.* Oakland, CA: New Harbinger Publications, Inc.

Deardorff, W. (2004). *The psychological management of chronic pain.* ContinuingEdCoursesNet: *www.continuingedcourses.net.*

Deardorff, W., & Reeves, J. (1997). *Preparing for surgery: A mind-body approach to enhance healing and recovery.* Oakland, CA: New Harbinger Publications, Inc.

Egoscue, P. (1998). *Pain free: A revolutionary method for stopping chronic pain.* New York, NY: Bantam.

Ford, N. (1994). *Painstoppers: The magic of all-natural pain relief.* West Nyack, NY: Parker.

Fuhr, A. (1995). Activator methods chiropractic technique: The science and art. *Today's Chiropractic*, July/August, 48–52.

Gorski, T. (2006). *Depression and relapse: A guide to recovery.* Independence, MO: Herald House/Independence Press.

Gorski, T., & Grinstead, S. (2006). *Denial management counseling workbook, revised.* Independence, MO: Herald House/Independence Press.

Gorski, T., & Grinstead, S. (2000). *Denial management counseling professional guide.* Independence, MO: Herald House/Independence Press.

Grant, M. (2005). *Pain control with EMDR: An information processing approach.* Submitted for publication.

Grinstead, S., Gorski, T., & Messier, J. (2006). *Denial management counseling for effective pain management.* Independence, MO: Herald House/Independence Press.

Grinstead, S., & Gorski, T. (2006). *Addiction-free pain management™: Relapse prevention counseling workbook, revised.* Independence, MO: Herald House/Independence Press.

Grinstead, S. (2002). *Addiction-free pain management™ recovery guide: Managing pain and medication in recovery.* Independence, MO: Herald House/Independence Press.

Grinstead, S., & Gorski, T. (1999). *Addiction-free pain management™: The professional guide.* Independence, MO: Herald House/Independence Press.

Khalsa, D., & Stauth, C. (2002). *Meditation as medicine: Activate the power of your natural healing force.* New York: Fireside.

Kennedy, J., & Crowley, T. (1990). Chronic pain and substance abuse: A pilot study of opioid maintenance. *Journal of Substance Abuse Treatment, 7*(4), 233–238.

Kingdon, R., Stanley, K., and Kizior, R. (1998). *Handbook for pain management.* Philadelphia, PA: W. B. Saunders.

Meade, T., et al. (1995). Randomized comparison of chiropractic and hospital outpatient management for low back pain: Results from extended follow-up. *British Medical Journal, 311,* 349–351.

Melzack, R., & Wall, P. (1965). Pain mechanisms: A new theory. *Science*, 150, 971–979.

Melzack, R., & Wall, P. (1982). *The challenge of pain.* New York: Basic Books.

Osterbauer, P., et al. (1992). Three-dimensional head kinetics and clinical outcome of patients with neck injury treated with manipulative therapy: A pilot study. *Journal of Manipulative Physiological Therapy*, 15(8), 501–511.

Pinsky, D., et al. (2004). *When painkillers become dangerous*. Center City, MN: Hazelden.

Reilly, R. (1993). *Living with pain: A new approach to the management of chronic pain*. Minneapolis: Deaconess.

Rogers, R., & McMillin, C. (1989). *The healing bond: Treating addictions in groups*. New York: W W Norton and Company.

Roy, R. (1992). *The social context of the chronic pain sufferer*. Toronto: University of Toronto Press.

Sarno, J. (1998). *The mind body prescription: Healing the body healing the pain*. New York: Warner Books.

Sarno, J. (1991). *Healing back pain: The mind body connection*. New York: Warner Books.

- *Useful Internet Resources*

Addiction-Free Pain Management™
http://www.addiction-free.com

Addiction-Free Pain Management™ describes the treatment system developed by Dr. Stephen F. Grinstead to help people suffering with chronic pain who also have coexisting addiction problems due to their prescription medication use.

Addiction No More
http://www.addictionnomore.com

Addiction No More offers drug and alcohol referrals to thousands of drug rehabilitation centers all over the United States and Canada.

American Academy of Pain Management
http://www.aapainmanage.org

The American Academy of Pain Management is the largest multidisciplinary pain society and largest physician-based pain society in the United States. The Academy is a nonprofit multidisciplinary credentialing society providing credentialing to practitioners in the area of pain management.

American Society of Addiction Medicine
http://www.asam.org

This medical specialty society is dedicated to educating physicians and improving the treatment of individuals suffering from alcoholism and other addictions, including those with pain and addiction.

American Society for Pain Management Nursing
http://www.aspmn.org

The American Society for Pain Management Nursing is an organization of professional nurses dedicated to promoting and providing optimal care of individuals with pain, including the management of its sequelae. This is accomplished through education, standards, advocacy, and research.

Body Mind Resources
http://www.bodymindresources.com

This site was founded to help keep people out of pain. Liam is a massage therapist and structural bodyworker with a mission to help and guide all those who are bold enough to begin the adventure of putting their bodies back together and getting out of pain.

Decision Maker® Institute
http://www.decisionmaker.com
This site is the home of several processes that enable people to make radical changes in their behavior and feelings by quickly and permanently eliminating the beliefs that determine what they do and feel. It also has techniques that de-condition the stimuli for such emotions as fear, anger, and guilt.

Drug Free at Last
http://www.drugfreeatlast.com/index.html
Selecting a drug rehab for yourself or someone you care about is one of the most important decisions you will make. On this site you can find the right treatment for drug abuse. Their services are free to the public. This site also includes valuable information about many of the drugs of abuse.

Enhanced Healing through Relaxation Music
http://www.enhancedhealing.com
On this site you will find relaxation music, positive affirmations, and online counseling for reducing stress and anxiety, promoting health, wellness, and healing, as well as improving self-esteem.

Gorski-CENAPS® Corporation
http://www.cenaps.com
This is the home site of Terence T. Gorski and the CENAPS® training team. Visit here for information on training and consultation services for recovery and relapse prevention issues for addiction and the related mental disorders, personality disorders, and lifestyle problems.

Holistic Help with Cynthia
http://www.holistichelp.net
On this site you will find sources for life management and support for people living with chronic illness, chronic pain, or disability. This site also offers education, consultation, pamphlets, articles, and e-books.

Jack Stem's Midwest Anesthesia Consultants
http://www.jackstem.com

Midwest Anesthesia Consultants is dedicated to providing current information to the professional healthcare provider as well as the consumer concerning anesthesia, conscious sedation, pain management, and nursing. By having current information, the provider and the consumer share in the benefits of better health care.

Metropolitan Pain Management Consultants
http://www.pain-mpmc.com

MPMC specializes in injuries and disease of the back such as work related injuries, persistent back pain before and after surgery, degenerative disc disease, spinal arthritis, disease of the facet joints, injury to muscles or ligaments, or pinched nerves in the neck and back. We treat complex regional pain syndrome (RSD), peripheral neuropathy, and pain associated with vascular conditions.

Mind Body Medical Institute
http://www.mbmi.org

The Mind/Body Medical Institute is a nonprofit scientific and educational organization dedicated to the study of mind/body interactions, including the relaxation response. This site offers online access to information from the world leader in the research and clinical practice of mind/body medicine.

Mind Publications
http://www.MindPub.com

This is a noncommercial, 24-7, self-help and coaching site to assist you with personal, family, and relationship problems such as anger, anxiety, depression, jealousy, marriage troubles, and parenting issues. It also offers help for coping with chronic illness or pain.

Mountain Health Pain Management
http://www.mountainhealthassociates.org

Mountain Health Associates is both a freestanding rural health family clinic and a pain management clinic. The clinics serve the greater Yuba-Sutter area of California, including but not limited to Yuba, Sutter, Colusa, and Butte counties.

The National Center for Complementary and Alternative Medicine (NCCAM)

http://nccam.nih.gov

NCCAM is dedicated to exploring complementary and alternative healing practices in the context of rigorous science; training complementary and alternative medicine (CAM) researchers; and disseminating authoritative information to the public and professionals.

National Fibromyalgia Association (NFA)

http://www.fmaware.org/index.html

The National Fibromyalgia Association (previously known as the National Fibromyalgia Awareness Campaign) is a "501(c) 3" nonprofit organization whose mission is to develop and execute programs dedicated to improving the quality of life for people with fibromyalgia.

NI-COR (Network International-Coalition for On-line Resources)

http://www.ni-cor.com

This site offers articles and directories for: health and wellness, addictions, prevention, recovery, medical terms, mental health, social issues, research, education, spirituality, and family.

Our Chronic Pain Mission

http://www.cpmission.com

This site offers support and information for a wide range of chronic pain, along with an "Ask Our Doctor" feature.

Prolothearpy

http://www.prolotherapy.org

This Web site offers a comprehensive description of the prolotherapy procedure as well as the many pain conditions that it effectively treats. The site also has a prolotherapist location search capability option as well as an interactive contact and questions function.

Scripps McDonald Center

http://mcdonald-center.scripps.org

Scripps McDonald Center is a nationally recognized organization dedicated to treating alcohol and drug abuse. The center provides a healing environment for people and their families needing help and receiving the tools and support they need to rebuild their lives.

Terence T. Gorski's Clinical Development
http://www.tgorski.com

Terry Gorski's Addiction and Clinical Development Web site is designed to keep decision makers, program managers, and clinicians up-to-the-minute on new developments regarding the Gorski-CENAPS® Model of Treatment.

Notes

Notes

Notes